More praise for *Getting to Calm*

"An ideal guide book for parenting teens, *Getting to Calm* shows how emotional intelligence starts in the home. Parents are given valuable strategies for managing their own emotions and tackling challenging situations, all with a keen focus on the critical importance of maintaining a strong parent-teen relationship. Indispensable!"

—**John Gottman, Ph.D.**
Author, *Raising an Emotionally Intelligent Child*

"This is a smart book. Filled with accessible science and illuminating stories, *Getting to Calm* offers sound advice for not only staying sane as a parent, but navigating the waters of your teen's life with clarity and skill so that both you and your adolescent will benefit. A wonderful contribution to every parent's library of support. Bravo!"

—**Daniel J. Siegel, M.D.**
Author, *The Mindful Brain: Reflection and Attunement
in the Cultivation of Well-Being, Parenting From the Inside Out*
and *Mindsight: The New Science of Personal Transformation*

"Required reading for parents who struggle with their teen. Here is true insight into the mental and emotional world of adolescents. Kastner and Wyatt offer parents useful, step-by-step tools for managing their own emotions in the face of teenaged chaos."

—**T. Berry Brazelton, M.D., and Joshua Sparrow, M.D.**
Harvard Medical School

Getting to
CALM

Cool-Headed Strategies for
Parenting Tweens + Teens

Laura S. Kastner, Ph.D.
Jennifer Wyatt, Ph.D.

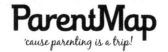

ParentMap is a Seattle-based resource for
award-winning parenting information.

parentmap.com

Printed in the United States of America
Published by ParentMap
Distributed by Ingram Publisher Services

02 08 20 10 KIN 01

Cover photograph: Alayne Sulkin
Cover design: Emily Johnson, Amy Chinn
Interior design and composition: Amy Chinn
Library of Congress Cataloging-in-Publication Data is available.

ISBN-13: 978-0-9823454-6-7
ISBN-10: 0-9823454-6-1

ParentMap dba Gracie Enterprises
7683 SE 27th St. PMB#190
Mercer Island, WA 98040
206-709-9026

ParentMap books are available at special discounts when purchased in bulk for premiums and sales promotions as well as for fundraisers or educational use. Place book orders at parentmap.com or 206-709-9026.

To our amazing children:
Cameron and Lindley
Megan, Molly, Andy and Jay

And the next generation:
Isaac, Julian and Maggie

Table of Contents

Preface to the Second Edition

Since the original publication of this book in 2009, the parenting landscape might appear to be a different place, as we look out on a world that is more diverse, more immersed in media, and—let's face it—more stressed out.

While the call for "cultural competence" has always been important, we now have a clearer view of the demographics that will comprise our increasingly diverse society. Young people who are comfortable working across different cultures and backgrounds will be more successful in jobs, careers, and in life.

Mobile media devices are omnipresent, and the impacts on all of us are both more highly scrutinized and hotly debated. Without question, media use has significant upsides, and it is also a powerful source of reward with addictive qualities. Families struggle to find ways to enjoy the benefits, resist the harms and protect family life from excess consumption. Some speculate that the new digital divide may be between families that give in to media use to the extent that it threatens their health and relationships and other families that manage use effectively. In these families, children receive the nourishment needed from optimal sleep, stay focused on homework and engage in activities and face-to-face relationships without media.

A third phenomenon, more widespread now than in 2009, is increased stress, stemming in large part from our fast-paced society. Like technology, stress is everywhere, and mental health problems are prevalent. Surveys shows that teens are more stressed than most parents realize. A value on basic mental health—on contentment, sleeping well, and lack of worry about present and future—is both undervalued and to be desired and cultivated.

Despite all that feels different, we find it gratifying as authors that the key messages in *Getting to Calm* remain sound. We have revised the chapters to include updated research and insights into changed circumstances. Nonetheless, the ability to self-calm and cope with adversity, as demonstrated in this book, is a more salient commodity than ever. Research continues to underscore the importance of emotional regulation and social-emotional intelligence. In the absence of a calm mindset, we aren't able to think, self-reflect, be aware of what's around us, and respond effectively. Having the skills to stay composed during hot parenting moments offers keen benefits, explored in this book. "Getting to calm" is still the biggest thing ever!

We are delighted to reissue the updated edition of this book with the enthusiastic, hard-working — and fun—team at ParentMap. It's extraordinarily satisfying to join forces with a group whose foremost goal is providing families with useful and trustworthy information. Sincerest thanks go to Alayne Sulkin, our dynamic and undaunted publisher, and all the staff who weighed in and championed this book including designer Amy Chinn and proofreader Elisabeth Kramer.

We'd also like to thank the moms, dads, and teens who contributed to this book by sharing their experiences — openly, humbly, and often with good humor. Although the family stories in each chapter are fictionalized composites, they've been created from real stories, most of them told to Laura Kastner anecdotally or in a clinical setting. We relied heavily on these families and remain inspired by them.

Our own families — parents, husbands, and children—supported and encouraged us every step of the way, unfailingly. We're so fortunate to have a couple of great and loving guys in our lives: Scott Wyatt and Philip Mease. And what would life be like without all the good friends who listened, counseled, and provided good cheer along the way?

Teen Difficulties Happen to the Best of Parents

Raising an adolescent is a daunting experience. Though parents love their tween or teen, and life together may go well most of the time, when our kids come across as bratty, defiant, thoughtless, or irresponsible, we can feel challenged like never before.

Very few of us sail through our children's adolescence completely unscathed, if not because of our teen's own actions, then because of a tricky situation, such as a social issue or a problem at school.

The good news is that most teens—especially those with caring, engaged, responsible parents—come out well-adjusted. Still, most families experience some complicated challenges stemming from their child's growing selfhood and push for independence. *Getting to Calm* breaks down 14 of the most frequently encountered and normal rough patches of adolescence, offering specific strategies for resolving these difficulties successfully and, better yet, for enhancing the teen's development in the process.

The concept of "getting to calm" is not merely about settling thorny situations, as desirable as that is for families. Rather, it pertains to an intentional mindset—tied to crucial discoveries about teen brain development and human emotions—that helps parents make good decisions and raise thriving teens. This book explains why the first step for effective parenting is "getting to calm," and includes techniques and approaches not only for achieving calmness, but for striking gold in the teen-parent relationship.

Neuro-imaging techniques developed over the last several decades have provided us with astounding discoveries regarding brain changes during adolescence. We now know, for example, that the emotional reactivity, impulsivity, and risk taking of the teen years are directly associated with the neural remodeling process that begins around 12 or 13 years of age. Technology has allowed us to track brain wiring and observe how the emotional centers of teens' brains can hijack their thinking process under certain circumstances.

Studies of the human brain can also illuminate why we adults may lose our tempers during volatile times when our kids push our buttons. Even with our fully mature brains, fear, anxiety, and anger can derail our reasoning skills and our best intentions to communicate effectively with our teens. Instead of dealing with teens under the influence of highly charged emotions—ours and theirs—we need to modify our approach and calmly access our "thinking" brains. In other words, we choose and deploy cool-headed strategies for connecting with, disciplining, and influencing our teens. Having high standards for teen conduct remains important, but parents who become informed about the teen brain and human emotions are in a stronger position to raise healthy, high-functioning tweens and teens.

Focusing on the parent-teen relationship, *Getting to Calm* includes a series of scripts that bring family realities to life. Side notes explain exactly why parents in some scripts make good moves that enhance relationships and effectiveness. Other parents head down the wrong road, and the notes clarify where and how these common mistakes occur. Getting to Calm weaves information about adolescent development and family dynamics with some of the latest findings on human biology to explain why teens do the things they do, why parents often trip up in their responses, and, in light of it all, how to bring out the best in teens and ourselves.

Getting to Calm is organized so that parents can turn to the material they need in a bad moment. Each chapter provides parents with the necessary tools to rectify a specific problem, but the process of achieving a calm mindset is best understood by reading this book from beginning to end.

It's also important to note what is not in this book. Some families will face severe turmoil and extremely tough problems with their teens, with issues such as depression, eating disorders, and substance addiction. Unlike the more typical 14 challenges covered in *Getting to Calm*, these disorders are clinical matters that require professional intervention. Likewise, there are vital issues that impact how we parent our children, such as culture, ethnicity, socio-economic status, and divorce. Crucial in determining any adolescent's experience and development, these highly complex issues can be better addressed by more specialized sources.

Though they may not always feel it, parents should be assured that they are important in their adolescent's life—and also more influential than their teen may ever let on. Nature provides teens with a built-in thrust for independence, which helps them become competent enough to leave the nest ultimately. But it also produces all the messy behaviors that are covered in *Getting to Calm*. These situations trigger intense interactions and moments when even the best of parents may lose their bearings.

As our children enter the teen years, most of us assume idealistically that if we are engaged, caring, and competent parents, our adolescents won't present us with any of the challenges mentioned in this book. But that's like wishing a toddler wouldn't fall while learning to walk or garbel pronunciation while learning to speak. Once we understand that growth and development involve a degree of messiness, we can put aside ego and misunderstanding and embrace the challenge of becoming effective and skillful parents.

Despite the occasional lapse, if we can operate from a place of calm most of the time, we are demonstrating to our teens the emotional skills they will need to be successful in their own lives. By "getting to calm," we are in a better position to choose the strategies that will see us through the toughest times of the tween and teen years. And most importantly, by staying level-headed, credible, and connected with our kids, we enhance a cherished relationship that holds families in good stead well beyond the teen years.

CHAPTER 1

When Your Sweet Child Morphs into a Sassy Teen

Why Are Today's Teens So Rude?

With open enthusiasm, a mom picks up her middle-school-age son and friends after soccer practice, offering them bagels as they pile into the car. "Nobody likes whole wheat" is all the "thank you" she gets from her son. Attributing his snippiness to low blood sugar, she wisely lets his little dig go. Besides, she's feeling good about herself as a mom. She has gone out of her way to get a healthy snack, and she's here for her son, despite her own crazy schedule.

The mom takes another stab at connecting, but in doing so resorts to a tired, overly general question destined to flop: "How was your day?"

"Fine," he says with a sigh of disgust.

Feeling deflated, she tries again by asking the time of his next soccer game. "Are you deaf?" the son snaps. "I already told you. I'm not telling you again."

Three for three. Here's a mom who has tried her best to tee up for a positive interaction with her son and is shot down each time. Crestfallen, she wonders whether she has done something wrong to be treated this rudely.

Has she?

Sometimes it sneaks up on parents little by little, and sometimes it happens in a flash: There's a difference in your relationship with your child. Maybe he's more impatient with you or she doesn't seem to want you around when she's with friends. Perhaps it's in the rolling of the eyes or the clamming up. Whatever the telltale sign, after a decade or so of being pretty good buddies most of the time, something has changed. And as with the mom in the soccer carpool, parents do little to trigger the new state of affairs.

Rudeness covers a broad range of behaviors that parents dislike, from argumentativeness to disgusted looks to blatant disrespect, and it's often a marker for profound changes ahead. Some parents wonder if they've lost their parenting touch. Trying to stay lighthearted, one mom described her daughter's transformation by saying, "Help! My child has been possessed by an alien!"

Making matters worse, most parents take the rudeness personally. It's hurtful, embarrassing, and appears to reflect bad character. Until adolescence, parents assume that if they're caring, loving, and consistent, their own sweet child won't morph into a shaggy, morose extraterrestrial. It happens anyway.

What's a parent to do? Above all, try to choose the right perspective, one born out of an accurate understanding of what's behind your child's rudeness. If you focus only on the dreadful manners and disrespect, you miss the dramatic thing they usually herald: the emerging of a new self, unrefined and uncouth as it is.

During the terrific and terrible twos, when toddlers are saying, "No, no, no!" parents aren't personally offended, because they realize that this assertiveness signals the inklings of an independent self. This is known as the "first autonomy phase." But during the "second autonomy phase" of the teen years (sometimes called "individuation"), the same rejection of parental dominance and authority can feel exquisitely personal and intended to trash everything we stand for. But that's the point: Reducing a parent's stature adds to the teen's own. As parents, we're the mighty oak trees. Only by cutting out some of our branches can our kids (seedlings) receive the light they need to become strong. Although true, this insight is small consolation to the parent suffering the damage.

Of course, teens don't spring forth at age 13 with a well-formed character and good, solid perspectives and values. The maturation of a self requires years of practicing and refining. Inevitably, through trial and error, teens will need to build skills of self-expression and self-assertion, and whom better to practice on than their parents? Parents experience being chopped down to size again and again, and it takes enormous perspective to see those moments as the hubbub of adolescent development, instead of a personal affront.

Even parents who understand this developmental stage wonder why teens are ruder today than a generation ago. Parents complain, "I never talked to my parents this way," and that's often true. Wanting our children to have good manners, we bristle at this trend and vow, "Not my child!"

Parents can get rudeness to stop, but not without a cost. Previous generations often prioritized obedience and propriety, and used tactics such as fear, threats, corporal punishment, and withdrawal of love to keep kids in line—essentially scaring them into submission. Parents who are intimidating and authoritarian will get less lip from their kids. The problem is that this domineering style of parenting doesn't lead to trust, security, or a long-term connection. It can also backfire, causing rebellion.

Like past generations of parents, we desire obedience, but we also put great value on connection, self-esteem, and communication. We don't want to be the scary person a teen would never turn to in a pinch.

You can have it both ways—with some careful finesse. If you want closeness and you want your teen to open up to you (at least occasionally), you have to be a reasonable, tolerant, and understanding parent, accepting of the thorny process of personal development. It's much easier to crack down: "Enough of that smart mouth. You're grounded for a month!" But if you're willing to put up with some rough spots, and if you play your cards right, you get something for what you suffer—a mutually trusting relationship.

Wouldn't it be great if parents could have a close relationship with their teens without contending with a degree of rudeness, bad attitude, and bratty behavior? Some can. An estimated 10 percent to 20 percent of teens report being happy most of the time.[1] Adolescence can be a relative cakewalk for families with teens who have mild temperaments and sunny dispositions. But for most of us, our children morph into more difficult and mysterious personalities during the teen years.

Staying Calm in the Face of Rudeness

The first thing a parent should do about rudeness is determine where it's coming from. Is it an overarching pattern born of an issue that needs special attention? Or is it a temporary phase—more a symptom of a teen's awkward, awakening self, showing itself as irritability and impatience? Remember, parents are privy to just a slice of their teen's behavior; what we see at home isn't the whole picture. Check in with teachers, coaches, and friends. Often parents hear from others how polite their teen is. Unless you're hearing about surliness or flippancy from everyone—including Grandma—you can't call it a pervasive behavior.

During adolescence, rudeness surfaces for so many reasons and out of so many sources that it seems an inevitable part of the age and stage. It's what you'll get if your teen is having a bad day, if you've frustrated them, if you've reminded them to do something, if you're imperfect, if they're stressed, or if you're just you and they're tired of it!

Since "Don't you dare talk to me that way!" is ultimately ineffective, what's the recourse for rudeness? Most families need a bag of tricks from which to pick and choose.

Here are a few possibilities:
- Ignore the rudeness.
- Address it directly, without threats or emotional flourishes, in clean language like "Cut it out."
- Don't give them what they want, but don't go on a guilt trip. Simply say something like "I don't feel inspired to take you to Kate's when you treat me this way." Stop there, let them have the last word, but don't take them to Kate's!
- Make a pre-emptive strike. For example, teens often show off in front of friends by being obnoxious to parents, so say something ahead of time

like "Yes, you can have Alex over, but I don't like it when you show off. Now you're on notice. Be respectful while he's here, or Alex will be sent home." With minor slippage, give a subtle warning, but be ready to follow through.

- Explain that their rudeness hurts your feelings with a comment like "Play back the tape of what just happened and see what you think. That was over the line and too mean." Express yourself in one or two sentences in objective language, again without guilt tripping. Don't do this often.

- Humor and wit can work wonders, if your timing is right. Although it wouldn't work for everyone, one mom made her point by responding to her daughter's relentless swiping at her younger sister with a convincing lion growl.

Whatever the approach, set your sights on what you need to accomplish. Perhaps, for example, you need to restrict media, set up a homework schedule, separate fighting siblings, or simply end an exchange that's spiraling downward. The important thing is to keep your mind on the goal—without being distracted by rudeness or bad manners.

The Tricky Issue of Manners

It's hard to trust that our teens may actually have manners when we don't see them. Manners and social graces instilled during childhood (such as respecting elders, behaving with civility, valuing good conduct) are still tucked inside most teens, but these behaviors often don't emerge, except in settings where they're anxious to look good and conform to adult expectations. All day at school, most teens work at restraining their impulses, being nice, and following rules, but around parents, they feel safer and more secure in letting their hair down. With puberty and other biological and emotional changes triggering the negative moods of adolescence, who better to "dump" these on than their secure base: their parents? The friction this causes helps a teen create distance, which in turn facilitates the process of becoming an individual, separate from parents and the previous identity of "child." Voilà! A teen is born.

But don't give up on manners entirely. Parents are absolutely entitled to some non-negotiable family protocol about how people are to be treated. The trick is to "pick your battles"—one of the wisest aphorisms known to parenting. Knowing when to weigh in—and with what rules—is key. For some families, it's no cell phones at the dinner table, while others care more about addressing other adults by their surnames. Choose carefully, since your target list at any moment has to be short. Imagine you're viewing a videotape of your last few hours with your teen. How much of the tape consists of nagging, lecturing, reminding, and badgering? If your negative remarks are creeping up and overshadowing your praise, humor, and positive overtures, then you're on your way to being blown off.

Because kids' temperaments differ wildly, background levels of negativity in the family will vary, too, regardless of parenting style. When life is already tilted a lot toward the negative with harder-to-parent kids (those with mood problems, attention deficit, defiant temperaments), it becomes nearly impossible to insist on the thank-you notes and keep a mostly positive relationship. Families with easier kids can insist on good manners, because they're not already bedeviled by all the work they're doing on big, pressing issues. It isn't fair, but sometimes we judge parents with well-mannered teens as better parents, when they're likely to have kids who are just easier to parent.

Family Story: **A Mom Deftly Handles a Defiant Teen**

Dee, a single parent of 16-year-old Maya and 9-year-old Aleisha, is in the kitchen making dinner and reminds her older daughter about sitting with her sister on Saturday night. Only the day before, Maya returned from overnight camp, where she was free as a summer's breeze from her family's customary expectations. Below is the story behind a mother-daughter tussle. This exchange shows a mom's keen discernment of which battle to pick. She lets a little attitude slide and sticks to her key goal of expecting compliance with a standing expectation, while deflecting other potential power struggles with masterful verbal aikido. The process comments explain the dynamics of the interchange and help us see how this mom figures out when to hold back.

Content *(what is said)*	Process *(underlying dynamics)*
Maya: You can't do this to me. You have to let me go out this Saturday. I've been at camp for two weeks! I need to catch up with my friends!	*The anguish of adjusting to home rules after being away is excruciating for Maya.*
Mom (Dee): Sorry, Maya . . . staying home with Aleisha on Saturdays is one of your family responsibilities, and I'm holding you to it.	*Mom determines that she had better be consistent with her rules, or else Maya will be rewarded for resisting her authority.*

Content *(what is said)*	Process *(underlying dynamics)*
Maya: Aleisha is so obnoxious when I sit with her. You have no idea, Mom. She ignores me. I can't get her to go to bed. If she is going to act like this, I don't think I should have to sit with her!	*Maya is angling for the upper hand by claiming hardship.*
Mom: We'll set you two down together for a talk after dinner.	*Mom tries deflection to shut down the argument.*
Maya: But Mom, it doesn't work. Last time I sat, she kept grabbing my phone and burping and singing.	*Maya keeps trying to engage Mom to talk about her sister's awful behavior.*
Mom: We've been here before, Maya. You have to limit the amount of time you talk on the phone when you sit. But let's back up here. Aleisha's behavior and the fact that you still have to stay home on Saturday night are two different . . .	*Mom almost goes for the bait, but stops short.*
Maya (interrupting): Isn't this Aleisha's night to set the table? You did it for her! That's not fair! She is so spoiled! You hold me to my chores, but not her! Why can't Aleisha just spend the night with a friend Saturday?	*Maya tries to get her mom on the defensive by pointing out her inconsistency. Maya then offers her a way out of the fight.*
Mom: Look, Maya. I'm not changing my mind. I know that you enjoyed a lot of freedom at camp, and coming home to business as usual around here is rough, but	*Mom stays on track, conveys her resolute position (to cue Maya to give up her protest), and offers Maya empathy for her understandable frustration.*

Content *(what is said)*	Process *(underlying dynamics)*
give it up. I'm sticking to our system. You get to go see your friends tonight anyway.	
Maya: I haven't seen my friends for such a long time, and they are probably planning something for Saturday night that will really be fun! You're not letting me have any social life! Plus, I'm the only kid I know who has to give up Saturday nights to take care of her sister.	*Maya detects that she is losing the battle, so she brings out the big guns: She is a victim to Mom's villainy, and no other kid has such a mean mom.*
Mom: I'm going to get dinner on.	*Mom doesn't bite the bait.*
Maya: You aren't listening to me! I thought good parents listen to their kids. You just don't care.	*As long as Maya is losing, she might as well punish mom by going for broke with the ultimate mommy put-downs. "Not listening" and "not caring" really means not caving.*
Mom: When we're settled down around here during the weekend, we can talk about chores again. But not now, with dinner ready, you all riled up, and my decision finalized about this Saturday. Let's get dinner on the table.	*Mom conveys her willingness to listen to Maya's feelings about chores when calm and non-reactive.*
Maya: You are so mean. This place is like a prison camp. I can't wait to go to college and get out of here.	*Since Maya is mad about the outcome of the fight, she wants to make mom "co-miserable" and suffer with her.*

Content *(what is said)*	Process *(underlying dynamics)*
Mom: Well, girl, I'm sure that college will be great for you. With all the practice you've had balancing fun with responsibilities, I'm sure you'll be able to handle the freedom of college very well indeed.	*Mom sees these last statements for what they are (last throes), and closes the fight down with a disarming compliment.*
Maya: I'm going to hate every minute of sitting.	*Mom knows that she'd better leave well enough alone. (Ending the fight is the priority. Having the last word isn't.)*

This argument could have been about anything—doing the dishes, using the car, making an expensive purchase. Too often, parents get wrapped up in specifics and who is more "right." By contrast, effective parents realize that what the tiff is "about" is less critical than managing the tug-of-war well. What are you like as you tell your teenager "yes" or "no"? Is there muscling for power? Aggressive shouting? Guilt tripping? Shaming? Lecturing? Complaining and then sudden caving? And an important question to ask yourself: Do you try to control more than you should?

A strong woman, Dee adheres to one of the basic premises of parenting: Control what you can control. Parents are well advised to focus on their own behavior and expectations for their teen, but not their teen's thoughts and feelings. Maya becomes defiant and even a little hostile to her mother, but Dee lets the saucy, disrespectful attitude go. She keeps her eye on the goal of getting Maya to honor her commitment, not for its own sake, but because she feels it necessary to reinforce family expectations.

Before yielding to our children's wants, we need to ask, "Whose interest is it in when I change my mind: my own, because I can no longer tolerate the barrage of negative emotions, or my child's, because there is some larger purpose to be served?" Though she took no enjoyment from her daughter's protest, Dee recognized the importance of remaining consistent. Otherwise, Maya might push for the same free rein the next weekend, and the battle could be even tougher. On the other hand, if Maya had respectfully requested to exchange Friday for Saturday night, for instance, or it was a special occasion, Dee could show more flexibility. But Maya is gunning randomly, at the last minute, and against the grain of the family rule.

Faced with Maya's accusations and criticism, Dee actively listens and shows empathy, but responds selectively. She stays positive by acknowledging her daughter's solid track record and suggesting that she'll be able to handle college. By introducing these positives, Dee short-circuits a reactive communication spiral. She also avoids humiliating her daughter—an ugly but common tactic for seizing the upper hand.

How is it that Dee is able to parent with such remarkable skill, wisdom, and good humor? Dee stays calm while under fire because she can separate her own thoughts and feelings from Maya's anger, distress, and distorted statements. At a deep level, Dee trusts her parenting instincts, in part because she is raising her children in much the same way she was raised. Reflecting on her own upbringing, she recalls having taken care of her brothers and sisters, and contributing to the household.

In a sense, each of us attended a kind of parenting school, and a very powerful one at that, based on the experiences we had growing up. When we become parents, we're likely to repeat many of the practices of our own upbringing, or, if we disagreed with them, perhaps swing to the other extreme. If generally comfortable with the way we were raised, we have a workable past to draw upon, and often feel more confident in our judgments. Parents who want to be significantly different from their own "family of origin" can struggle, because they often second-guess the instincts guiding their decisions and judgments. Regardless of a parent's background, the following guidelines for "authoritative parenting" show parents how to steer a calm course.

The Most Effective Parenting Style for Raising a Successful Teen

Dee's interactions with Maya illustrate the qualities of "the authoritative parent," one of three basic parenting styles. Trends in childrearing come and go, but the value of authoritative parenting has been well established through research that has held up for decades.[2] Authoritative parents—unlike "permissive" or "authoritarian" parents—raise kids who are socially and emotionally competent, have high self-esteem, and are capable and independent.

Permissive . . . **AUTHORITATIVE** . . . Authoritarian

These parents possess three all-important qualities: thoughtful control, high warmth, and effective communication.

Quality 1: Thoughtful Control. On a continuum, authoritative parents are midpoint between permissive and authoritarian parents.

Low control . . . THOUGHTFUL CONTROL . . . Excessive control

Permissive parents routinely cave to their teens' desires and weaken when faced with their teens' defiance. Though involvement with their children varies (some are overly involved and others are disengaged), their key feature is that they lack real authority and don't effectively set limits or discipline their children. Some of these parents genuinely believe that children should have few limits, but many more are desperate to avoid conflict.

Permissive parents can end up explaining, defending, and reasoning with their children so much that limits and family policies fall by the wayside. An important distinction: Permissiveness and flexibility are not synonymous. Flexibility is a positive trait in parents; it's the ability to adapt to changing circumstances and the changing needs of their children as they grow and mature.

At the opposite pole are authoritarian parents—"give/go" parents. ("I give the order, you go do it!") Not interested in dialogue, negotiation, or the feelings of their teens, they tend to adhere to a rigid set of standards. Authoritarian parents may defend their tyrannical positions by raising principles of discipline and accountability, but often they are reactive people who don't have the patience for mutual exchange of thoughts and feelings. Adolescents can ensnare them in unprecedented power struggles. When a parent commands a teen, "Do it or else!" some teens will actually leap for the "or else" out of indignation, pride, and a desire to assert the new self.

Between the two extremes is the authoritative parent, who exercises control judiciously—to teach, guide, and support—rather than as an assertion of power for its own sake. Shrewd choosers, authoritative parents know when to flex. Allowing their children to weigh in to some degree with their preferences, such parents use their authority when and where it matters, mixing it with warm and effective communication to establish trusting relationships. They pick their battles, based on parenting rule no. 1: Keep a mostly positive relationship. A useful standard is five to one: Each negative interaction needs to be balanced with five positive ones.

Quality 2: High Warmth. Warmth, as measured decades ago in original research on parenting types, pertains to qualities now described as "secure attachment" and "parent-child connectedness." Optimally, children feel accepted for exactly who they are, even while parents create expectations of greater maturity and improved habits. Beginning in early infancy, parents who are responsive and attuned to their child year after year develop a trusting, secure bond with them. A strong parent-child connection means that the child can count on his parents' love and support through thick and thin, and even through the inevitable messiness of the teen years. Strong parent-child connectedness has also been shown to be predictive of lower levels of substance use, teen pregnancy, and school problems.[3]

Cold and disengaged . . . **WARM** . . . Enmeshed
APPROPRIATELY ENGAGED

On a continuum, warm parents are found midpoint between disengaged parents, who have neither empathy for their children's feelings nor a grasp of their developmental needs, and enmeshed parents, whose emotional lives are fused with those of their children.

Quality 3: Effective Communication. Effective communication means that each person's needs, desires, and opinions are considered. Teens need to know that their parents respect them and incorporate their ideas and opinions when possible. Not that we always agree and approve, but we're willing to listen and empathize with their position, especially when the exchange is appropriate and respectful. Sometimes effective communication involves staying quiet and conveying support through body language.

Communication cutoff . . . **EFFECTIVE** . . . Unbounded talk
COMMUNICATION

Effective communication is the happy medium between shutting down all teen input and feedback and unbounded talk. Unbounded talk is unfiltered, with parents responding to every challenge, complaint, and accusation a teen throws out.

Cutting off communication sends a message that the teen's feelings and views will not be heeded, now or ever, and the parent's views and needs are the only ones that matter. As tempting as it may be to shut down a surly teen complaining about "stupid" homework or a "boring" relative, there's a clear downside to minimizing or trying to control negative feelings. Research on school-age children shows that children whose parents dismiss and disapprove of their negative expressions end up less resilient, less socially skilled, and less capable in school.[4]

Effective communication supports a teen's need for autonomy. Whether it's a bid for new privileges or a challenge to our values, teens would not develop the competencies they need to lead independent lives without testing their thoughts and new skills. A healthy exchange of ideas and validation of teens' feelings are building blocks of closeness, trust, and mutual understanding. Parents who respectfully listen to their teens' beliefs and ideas, even if they disagree with them, are more likely to have high-functioning teens.

Just as authoritarianism was an adverse trend of previous generations, excessive talking has become a crutch for some of today's parents. Uncomfortable with authority and afraid of angering their child by making unpopular decisions, permissive parents often stay engaged in negative exchanges, defending and rebutting all the distorted accusations teens make, particularly when they're cranked up. When a teen (or parent) is out of control emotionally, the parent should end this kind of discussion with a promise to hear the teen's concerns at a calmer moment. Parents who persist in arguing have themselves to blame when their teen loses it with a "F--- you." The wise parent knows that productive communication cannot occur while either party is highly emotional.

The best exchanges are calm and respectful. They may happen over a backrub late at night, in a carpool—whenever kids and their parents are in a good, neutral, or contemplative mood. Parents can usually sense those moments when talking is going well, and they're golden.

———————————————

One of the big deep secrets of childrearing is that sometimes our kids will dislike us intensely. During adolescence, it can sometimes feel like outright loathing, even in healthy, loving families. If we've been intentional and conscientious in our parenting, we can tolerate our teen's rudeness and disdain, knowing that it is temporary and only one part of our relationship. Self-trust, wisdom in picking battles, and an inner dialogue of affirmation (of self and teen) have to keep us going during lapses of rapport. And for the teen with a challenging temperament (moodiness, attention deficit, defiance), these lapses may be frequent, intense, and sometimes all but unbearable. Parents of these teens need a lot of cheerleading and encouragement from well-informed spouses, friends, and sometimes professionals, because of all the emotion such teens have to dump on even a very good parent.

Raising a teen is a long-term process, and, like any construction project, it's messy. Parents who understand that the rudeness and disrespect are part of the underpinnings of building a self will see the folly of trying to control it all and will focus on controlling what they can control—their own moves and reasonable expectations for teen conduct—and not the teen's occasional negative thoughts, feelings, and mouthiness.

Sometimes damage control is all you can expect in a difficult situation. If you've stayed calm and haven't added fuel to the flames, you've done your best, because you've kept your own negativity out of the mix. Rudeness and bad attitudes are more about forming a self than most parents realize. They relate to hormones, brain development, and the urge to draw close to peers and away from parents who have what feels like interminable demands, unreasonable expectations, and irritating personalities. Building a self takes a long time. It's an untidy process, and it's miraculous.

CHAPTER 2

When Smart Teens Do Really Dumb Things

When—and Why—Teens Don't Use Their Heads

Example one: It was the proverbial dark and stormy winter night, and a ninth-grade girl "disappears" during the break of her evening basketball practice. Alarmed, the coach contacts her parents and stops practice to mount a search. Mom begins making phone calls to her daughter's friends, while dad heads out in the car to patrol the area around the school. An hour later, they find her in the shadow of a nearby building, laughing and chatting with her new boyfriend. Her parents are furious at her self-indulgence and inability to see the impact of her behavior on many others.

Example two: Not only has this eighth-grader been repeatedly reminded about his after-school orthodontist appointment, he also has a sticky note with the information in a highly visible place in his backpack. But no sooner is he out the school door than a friend says, "I'm starved. Let's catch the bus and get some tacos." When his mom receives the "no show" call from the orthodontist, she's steaming and goes after her son for being irresponsible and blowing off an important appointment.

Example three: Parents learn through school that their daughter posted photos on Instagram of girls in their underwear at her sleepover, which someone then photoshopped into naked poses and transmitted digitally throughout the school body. Because of child pornography implications, legal authorities are consulting with the school. Although the parents know that antics like this at sleepovers are "normal," they have talked about careful posting numerous times and can't believe the stupidity of her post—and how serious the repercussions might be.

Example four: A group of high school boys are playfully roughhousing outside school, teasing and jostling one another. Along comes a boy known for his studious ways, and as he walks by, one of the boys impulsively sticks out his foot and trips him, causing him to fall and fracture his wrist. School authorities describe the boy's rowdy action as malicious and mean-spirited.

To these behaviors and countless more like them, the classic parent response is "What were you thinking? I raised you better than this!" It's a rare parent of an adolescent who hasn't been frustrated, if not infuriated, at some mindless teen move, and because the teen really should know better by now, the parent judges him as deliberately thoughtless and irresponsible—or worse. When stupid behaviors multiply, it can start to look like a defect in a child's character. Though the teens in the examples may be somewhat guilty as charged, something else rather startling and profound is unfolding that may mitigate their offenses.

Extraordinary Discoveries in Brain Science

Brain-imaging studies have changed our understanding of adolescence, as we reassess what's behind the recklessness, thoughtlessness, and carelessness of teens. Behaviors once attributed to raging hormones or self-centeredness now appear also to be tied to brain development during adolescence. Research in this area suggests that quite often teens aren't intentionally making bad choices and decisions. Rather, under certain circumstances, there may be no real decision-making happening at all—particularly when they're excited and hyped up.

Studying the brains of normal teens as they grow, researchers discovered that a massive reorganization of the brain gets under way starting around 11 or 12 years of age.[1] Known as the reasoning part of the brain, the prefrontal cortex undergoes reconstruction in a process often characterized as "pruning and blossoming." Likened to a CEO, the prefrontal cortex oversees "executive thinking functions," such as planning ahead, making informed judgments, and weighing the costs, benefits, and risks of various decisions. In the adolescent brain, almost half of the existing synapses (connections between brain cells) are whittled away in this critical area for thinking, as new connections are being rewired and the brain is ramping up to become faster and more efficient once the process is completed.

What does all this mean to parents? The dramatic reconfiguration of the prefrontal cortex during adolescence signals increased opportunity as well as increased vulnerability for the teen, both of which have direct bearing on how we can better parent teens.

Teens are vulnerable because just when their independent spirits render them in need of good judgment skills, they're literally losing parts of their minds! And most importantly, their impulse-control networks are not fully developed until age 22 for females and 25 for males. Because it takes a quarter of a century for our children's full mental capacity to reach maturation, they often do need their parents to think with them and sometimes for them.

Moreover, compared to adults, teens are extra sensitive to dopamine, the neuro-chemical in our brain that is released in anticipation of rewards. These rewards could include sex, substances, food, media, retail items, or just about anything that shouts "goody!" to an individual's brain. The problem here is clear: teens are *more* drawn to "goodies" but have *less* impulse-control capacity. And therein lies the recipe for a lot of dumb mistakes.

On the flip side is increased opportunity. In the simplest sense, this boils down to "use it or lose it." During adolescence, the brain becomes more specialized through a process of elimination, sloughing off unnecessary neural branches and forging stronger connections based on how the brain is used. Essentially, the neurons that fire together are wired together. The neurons that fire as teens are reading, practicing piano, or playing soccer are forming new neural connections. Enriching activities like these enhance teens' lives, but so does the independence to make mistakes and learn from them, as the thicket of neurons is pruned into a well-manicured, blooming garden.

As we've always believed but can now actually see in the brain, adolescence is a critical time for learning and growth. That's why we don't want our teens sitting in front of an electronic screen all day. We also don't want them focused solely on academics. The prefrontal cortex is wired into the limbic system, the emotional part of the brain that helps us make sense of the world and relate to others. Intricately linked, emotions inform intellectual reasoning, and vice versa. Teens need to be interacting with people to develop social skills. They need to be out in the world, engaging in a mix of extracurricular activities, and coping with and solving a range of problems. And they need time to reflect and make sense of their experiences, particularly in our hurry-up American culture.

The increased opportunity for learning associated with the reconfiguration of the adolescent brain is exciting news. The increased vulnerability, on the other hand, is a more frightening prospect, because it puts all teens at risk when impulses and dangerous circumstances converge.

Why Emotion Often Overrides Reason in Teens

One side effect of the major revamping of a teen's prefrontal cortex is that thinking processes are easily thrown off course. Neural paths for reasoning, judgment, and inhibiting impulses have yet to be fully established, and activity is triggered in the emotional parts of the brain more readily and more often.

In the center of the emotional brain is a small, almond-shaped organ called the amygdala. Whether in relation to stage fright, a family fight, or a rude encounter with a friend, the amygdala often determines our response to distressing or frightening circumstances, causing us to "fight, flee, or freeze." It dictates our impulsive reactions, such as jumping out of the way of a snake without conscious thought. Adolescents are vulnerable to what is called "amygdala hijacking," meaning that instead of using their "thinking" prefrontal cortex in the same way as adults, neural impulses are stimulated in the amygdala, particularly during arousing and exciting situations.

Interesting research in this area illustrates how teens misread signs of emotion.[2] Shown a face, teens were found to mistake looks of fear and surprise as anger and hostility. Brain images revealed that the emotional parts of their brains were lighting up during this test, indicating that they were using this part of the brain to decode the facial expression. Adults using their prefrontal cortex will recognize that the face is registering surprise. No wonder teens accuse their parents of being "angry" so often! Hanging out in their emotional brain, teens don't read our concerns accurately—they just think we're mad at them.

Simply put, the prefrontal cortex in teens has not yet developed to the point that it can rein in the intense reactions of the emotional part of their brains that's screaming, "I want what I want!" Adults experience the same phenomenon when they're overwhelmed by anger, anxiety, or craving, but for teens, it's true much more of the time.

These and other astonishing discoveries about brain development go a long way toward explaining why really good kids with really good parents will still experience tough times during adolescence. Some teens are more prone than others to go bonkers, because individual personalities and temperaments are a big factor, as are parenting and circumstances. Nonetheless, though we supply our teens with education and information, warning them of risks and consequences, they can toss it all to the wind when they are riled up and ruled by their "emotional brains."

The risks inherent to the teen years have been characterized by neuroscientists as "big engine, poor driving skills, faulty brakes, and high-octane gas." The big engine refers to the brash new push for autonomy teens are attempting; poor driving skills result from the reconstruction of teens' prefrontal cortexes and the emotional hijacking that ensues; faulty brakes describe teens' lack of impulse control; and high-octane gas refers to the intense emotions accompanying adolescent hormonal changes. The amygdala has receptor sites for testosterone, and, by the end of puberty, testosterone can increase by an astonishing 1,000 percent in boys and more than 20 percent in girls. As a result of hormonal fluctuations, boys will charge ahead with more intensity, passion, aggression, territoriality, and confidence. With their amygdalae overstimulated by testosterone, boys have been shown to seek novelty and stimulation.[3] With the effects of estrogen, girls—no surprise—can have greater emotionality.

Ages 5 to 11 can be relatively smooth for parents. With the right supervision and guidance, most youngsters can be conditioned to follow rules. "Mom said I could go around the block, but not across the street," they'll repeat to themselves. Young kids can have poor impulse control, and they will break rules, but they're more attuned to their parents' direction, and most want parental approval more than fights over independence. Before puberty, children typically lack the urge, the energy, and the drive for the kind of thrill-seeking that's characteristic of teens.

Some children are born with a novelty-seeking personality that becomes evident in early childhood: "He's headed down the hill backward on a tricycle, going full speed with hands in the air!" When these kids undergo the brain changes of adolescence, it's double trouble. Their parents can be supremely discouraged by one dumb teen move after another, even though the predicament is completely built in biologically. These parents deserve awards for surviving adolescence with relationships and wits intact. Between the challenges of temperament and brain development, daily life can be a rollercoaster, as illustrated in the following story.

Family Story: A Teen's Big Blunder Triggers Extreme Parent Reactions

Temperamentally, 15-year-old Terry Desanto has the high energy, self-confidence, and impetuousness of a young buck. Popular, athletic, and smart, he specializes in mischief-making—stomping on ketchup packets in the school cafeteria, coating door knobs with salve, sneaking out at night to "TP" houses. Terry's most extreme prank, an act of vandalism, occurred on the evening before his high school's state basketball playoffs. Egged on by a group of guys who remained outside the school, Terry and a friend, Sam, slid through a gym window and spray-painted racy, provocative slurs against the opposing team on the gym walls.

The next morning, mobs of students crowded into the gym to see the graffiti. Classes were disrupted, tests had to be postponed, and a special janitorial staff was called in. Ultimately, the principal discovered the culprits and suspended Terry and Sam from school for a week. Donna, Terry's mom, has done her best to rein in her wild son, but her reaction to the news shows her lapse in a stressful moment.

Content *(what is said)*	Process *(underlying dynamics)*
Mom (Donna): How do you think I feel being the mom with the kid who always gets in trouble? Your behavior thoroughly humiliates me! I can't go anywhere without someone asking me about your latest shenanigans. This mess is the ultimate! This is vandalism! You've defaced school property!	*Emotionally aroused, Mom shouts accusations and focuses on her own humiliation. She doesn't see that she has put herself in the spotlight. The heat should be on Terry and getting him to critique his own actions.*

Content *(what is said)*	Process *(underlying dynamics)*
Terry: Don't get hysterical, Mom. It was only spray paint. It's not like it's permanent. Graffiti is all over our school anyway.	*A common defense to any extreme misdeed is minimization.*
Mom: I can't believe you're downplaying this! Don't you realize you could get expelled, not just suspended, for this! Do you know where you're headed with behavior like this?	*One type of power struggle occurs when one person claims crisis and the other counterbalances through resistance. The result is mutual anger and no productive outcome.*
Terry: Chill out, Mom! God, you should see your eyes—they look like they are about to pop out! You act like I'm an axe murderer or something!	*Although Terry is 100 percent guilty of his crime, his mother's approach continues to call attention to her emotion rather than his misdeed.*
Mom: Terry, I swear, I don't know what I'm going to do with you. You can't get out of this one. This one is big, really big.	*Mom is deflated by Terry's tactical move to side-step his guilt by stating that he is not guilty of murder.*
Terry: Mom, you know the principal has it in for me. She calls you all the time about stupid stuff. Sam was the one with the idea, and I'm getting all the blame. Other guys were hanging around rooting us on.	*Once Terry sees that Mom has run out of steam a bit, he redirects her attention skillfully to shared blame and to his being made a scapegoat.*
Mom: Well, that's true. You mean the principal believes that you are the mastermind?	*Mom bites the bait, desperately wanting some relief from the idea that her son (and their family) is singled out as "bad" at the school.*

At this point, Donna phones the principal for further information about the incident and an explanation for why other boys cheering on Terry and Sam were not punished. When the principal reiterates her position, Donna accuses her of having it in for her kid. After hanging up, Donna is not only angry, she's embarrassed about having lost it with a school authority.

Desperate for support, Donna phones Sam's mother, who likewise targets Terry as the main instigator. Donna realizes she needs to cool off and involve her husband, Ray. Like all people, they have inclinations and tend to react in predictable patterns. Donna knows that if she comes on too strong, Ray will soft-pedal and defend Terry. Initially, Donna stays calm as she briefs Ray, but soon ingrained patterns re-emerge.

Content *(what is said)*	Process *(underlying dynamics)*
Dad (Ray): Terry, you showed horrible judgment in pulling this prank. You're going to be totally grounded for a month and banned from contact with Sam until further notice.	*Dad is very upset about Terry's crime and knows that he should move quickly to sanction Terry so he gets credit for staying firm on discipline.*
Terry: OK, Dad, but you gotta at least let me go to the game. These are the playoffs, and since I can't play, I need to be there to support the team. I'll just sit with you. It's punishment enough that I can't play.	*Dad loves these games almost as much as his son. He feels himself weakening. Maybe his son has a point. He wonders whether his wife will accept that the rest is sufficient punishment.*
Dad: Well, I don't know.	*Dad becomes tongue-tied.*
Mom (Donna): NO WAY! This has got to stop. Today he's spraying gym walls; tomorrow he'll be calling in bomb scares.	*Mom feels betrayed by Terry, the school, Sam's mom, and now, her husband. His softening makes him the perfect target for her rage, fear, and helplessness.*
Dad: Now, Donna, aren't you getting a little carried away?	*The best defense is often a misplaced offense: Dad defends his*

Content *(what is said)*	Process *(underlying dynamics)*
You're acting like he's a juvenile delinquent.	*son and gets off the hot seat for his potential softening on the discipline by doing what Terry did earlier— focusing on mom's exaggerated indictment of Terry's character.*
Mom: How dare you "Now, Donna" me! What audacity! You never get the phone calls. I'm constantly humiliated while you stay safely hidden in your office. These pranks are so male! You encourage Terry by telling your stories about your fraternity antics! Don't you see how you indirectly encourage him?	*Parental mutual blaming has essentially gotten Terry off the hook for now. High anxiety has brought out many of these family members' worst habits—polarizing, deflecting blame, extreme thinking, criticizing, and ineffective problem-solving.*

The Desantos feel overwhelmed by Terry's high-energy temperament, excitability, and lack of self-control. Beleaguered by constantly dealing with his shenanigans and insolence, they lose patience and focus, the situation goes south, and Terry gets off the hot seat. This dynamic has become a well-practiced dance within the family: Terry has learned how to "get his parents' goats" by denying and minimizing, which helps create the fray that keeps him from facing his wrongdoing in a meaningful way. To their credit, Dad tries to be the hard guy, while Mom tries to keep her grip. But anxiety and high emotion get the better of them and push them into their typical pigeonholes of Mom overreacting and Dad compensating in order to cool things off, with Terry stirring the pot all the while. The result is a very bad moment in a good family's year, related to two circumstances: Terry's immature brain plus an inadequate parent response. What might they have done instead? Some suggestions follow.

Helping Kids Learn From Their Mistakes

Teens should never get off the hook for their dumb moves. But now that we know how easily they default to their emotional brain and act in the moment, we should take care not to leap to harsh assumptions and treat them as if they're one notch up from hardened criminals. The question isn't: "Did he think he was going to get away with this?" It's: "Did he think at all?" For the petty pranks and rash actions of many teens, the problem lies in their brains, not their moral fiber. Typically, teens lack a full up-and-running thinking brain to guide them well in times of excitement. Even when there's real cause for discouragement, parents need to hang in there with their teen to try to build an understanding of the impact of their actions. This kind of moral fiber is developed through many patient, well-guided briefing sessions after many teen mistakes. Some steps in this process follow.

Start by presenting what you know as calmly as possible to see what they say. Edit out a huge amount of what you feel and avoid shaming, blaming, moral outrage, and indignation. Like kids of all ages, teens are likely to be nervous under fire and try to cover up. Stay composed when they start to dig in and deny, so that you aren't diverting the attention to yourself or arousing them even more. This approach isn't about being nice. It's calculated to set up the situation so that their brains are calm enough to connect the dots and see where they went wrong.

Be on guard for moves—theirs and yours—that can escalate conflict. Even when parents are 100 percent right, if we come in lecturing on a high horse, our teens feel accused and provoked, and will probably fight back. Only too easily do teens become hot-headed and defensive. Before you know it, the tables will turn, and your sound wisdom will be wasted. Don't take the bait and be sidetracked by extraneous information (other participants, history, extenuating circumstances). And beware of any teen's ability to drive a wedge between parents!

If a teen shows no sign of being remorseful and tries to minimize his actions, counterattack, or divide parents, take a break. It is never in a parent's self-interest to keep any type of deteriorating power struggle alive, because it will always get worse. Don't be pressured by your teen's wrong-headedness and insolence into feeling you have to slam back. It's always the parent's job to maintain control of the situation. Discipline can wait until everyone is calm and able to use the thinking brain. If your teen clams up, state your piece succinctly and pursue a "carrot and stick" approach.

Use a "carrot and stick" approach to encourage self-reflection. Think about what discipline is supposed to accomplish. The word "discipline" derives from the Latin word discere, which means learning. The big goal is for teens to examine their own behavior in a thoughtful way, see where they went wrong, and sort out how to do things differently next time. Tell them outright, "Whatever we decide in terms of consequences, it will be better for you if we can see that you're capable of learning from this disaster." Stay serious and calm. Let them know that it is in their best interest to demonstrate an understanding of the problem, because discipline will be based on their level of insight and ability to self-critique and make amends. Then be more lenient or severe, depending on what they eke out.

Use techniques that will allow them to see where they went off track and will ultimately build connections in their thinking brain. When the time is right, have a debriefing session. Parents can ask neutral questions and let the teen fill in the blanks with their own analysis. Good questions to weave into your talk might include: "What happened?" "What threw you off course?" "Did you ever have any second thoughts?" "What kept you from paying attention to them?" "What would you do differently next time?" Debriefing is the teen's opportunity to figure out how the disaster unfolded step by step, identify where he went off track, and determine how he might have self-corrected. Think about ways to increase teens' empathy for people they've impacted. And since teens tend to clam up, encourage even the smallest signs of remorse and build on them.

Writing about the incident can be a great technique, because it stimulates teens' thinking. Teens can write amazing reflections once they've recovered from the crisis and are in a more thoughtful state of mind.

If parents are mild tempered and the teen continues to make light of wrongdoing, the parents should raise the volume to get their child's attention. During a crisis, most parents need to guard against complicating the emotional field by dumping out too many feelings and overwhelming the teen with guilt and shame. Other parents who are gentle and soft-spoken may actually have to make an effort to dial it up in order to put sufficient heat on the teen. This can occur in the context of a great relationship, with nice parents and nice teens who rarely scuffle. Turning up the volume becomes an opportunity for parents to target a problem behavior. In general, the gravity of tone needs to match the seriousness of the crime.

Consider seeking professional advice if you feel stuck. Through a calm debriefing session, most parents can engage in a process to help teens understand where they went wrong and make reparations. A well-handled crisis can be a fantastic learning experience. If parents have been using all the right techniques (above) and teens are still refusing to take responsibility, it's probably time to raise the level of response, particularly with serious infractions (driving under the influence, shoplifting, vandalism) or repeat offenders. In this situation, a professional consultation may be the big gun needed to impress upon the teen the seriousness of the offense.

The Myth of Immunity

For decades, the term "myth of immunity" or "invincibility" has been used to describe how teens deny danger, believing nothing bad will happen to them. Although teens may be able to cite various health facts associated with dangerous behaviors (drinking and driving or unprotected sex, for example) their actions on Saturday night seem to say, "These risks don't apply to me—I'm special." Historically, this bravado has been attributed to teens' hormones or egocentric style. We have now learned that their brain maturation process, in conjunction with the changes of puberty, accounts for their shortsightedness and poor judgment. In the heat of the moment, teens don't have the mental equipment to identify the negative consequences of egging a neighbor's car or—a more frightening scenario—speeding down a highway. It's the "big engine, poor driving skills, faulty brakes, and high-octane gas" that put them in jeopardy and is behind much of teen mortality.

The myth of immunity doesn't apply across the board, of course. Teens who are thrill-seekers or have attention deficit disorder (ADD) are more prone to impulse, putting themselves more readily in peril. Teens who are anxious, shy, or avoidant tend to hold themselves back and will steer themselves away from risky or arousing situations. Whatever the temperament, the best time for parents to access their teen's thinking brain is when they're calm—perhaps at night as they're getting ready to go to sleep, or during a car ride.

Parenting a teen involves lots of supervising from near and afar, limiting risks, and knowing hot spots (such as any place where there's a swirling mass of peers!) to oversee with extra vigilance. Every teen needs to have fun and experience independence. With thrill-seeking kids, parents need to be more clever in lining up safe places (extracurricular activities, camps, sports) where it's possible to harness the wild side and keep their teens from harm.

When smart teens do really dumb things, parents can engage in very effective discipline, but does that mean teens can use what they've learned on every future Saturday night? Probably not. They'll be living in their emotional brain for years. With many teens, a good debriefing and a short leash following a crisis will keep them mindful and remorseful for a few months at most. Right when everyone relaxes, teens can be back at it with another lark, risky adventure, or lapse in judgment when excited or hanging with their herd. But the good part of this whole untidy process is that learning is taking place, as the memory part of the emotional brain links up increasing numbers of neural connections with the thinking brain. This process, along with a supportive home life throughout the teen years, enhances reasoning and emotional intelligence for the rest of their lives.

The goal for parents is to do the best they can with each experience. We can't rush brain development. Building connections and understanding is a cumulative process and will take years. Simply put, don't expect one-trial learning and don't give up on your teen.

During the teen years, young people become capable of dazzling and sophisticated hypothetical thinking. Able to grasp symbolic logic, they can perform abstract mathematics and compose impressive essays on truth and beauty and right versus wrong. Despite classroom smarts and the common sense they show during close conversations, their good minds can be lost to them under certain circumstances. When adolescents are caught up in situations that rile them, their thinking is hijacked by their emotional brain; their prefrontal cortex remains insufficiently developed to step in and overrule; and they do things they were told never to do, not so much deliberately but without truly thinking at all.

Parents who become aware of adolescent brain development can feel less injured when their good kid does a bad thing and less inclined to severe judgments of their teen and themselves. In the midst of a teen calamity, angry parents may resort to lecturing and punishing, which typically revs up a teen's emotional brain and renders them less capable of self-analysis. Disciplinary action remains important, but the best vehicle for it is a well-handled debriefing session. This technique allows teens to critique themselves, examine where they went astray, and develop their thinking brains.

For all of the headaches and heartaches tied to brain development during adolescence, there is much that's remarkable and exciting about this reconfiguration process. Opportunities for learning abound, as old neural connections are sloughed off and new ones are rapidly formed. Teens' growing brains are highly adaptable to the new; note, for example, how they can run rings around most parents with new technology. Teen musicians lay down the neural circuitry for muscle memory; chess players pick up moves they've seen without really memorizing them; and teens adept at building things solve construction problems intuitively. Whenever parents feel disheartened or discouraged by the lapses of reasoning, motivation, and judgment intrinsic to adolescent brain development, they can remind themselves of the flip side of the process and the plenitude of new skills and talents blossoming during these years.

Engaging and iconoclastic members of our society, adolescents are capable of great leaps of creativity and spontaneity. Living in their emotional brains, they naturally think outside the box. One can suppose that because it takes so little effort to unhinge their thinking brains, they're freer to abandon themselves to daring acts of athleticism, not to mention acts of bravery. Brain development explains why teens are so quick to try new things and forge into the unknown, but it also explains why they still need their parents.

CHAPTER 3

When Your Trustworthy Teen Pulls a Fast One

Family Story: Skillful Handling of a Teen Crisis

Pleasant news rarely comes in the form of a late-evening phone call. Stella has just learned from another parent that her conscientious 17-year-old son, Chris, has deliberately deceived her. It feels like a punch in the stomach. In her mind, she replays how nonchalantly Chris had told her he was sleeping over at Jason's, when he had every intention of heading to a concert hours away and camping out with a bunch of friends. "He's never done anything like this," she thinks. "How could he have pulled the wool over my eyes so cleverly? What else is he up to that I don't know about?"

To make matters worse, Stella's husband is out of town, leaving her alone to fume. Knowing that Chris and the other boys arrived safely at the concert does little to calm her mushrooming anger—anger at her son's blatant lie and anger at herself for being naïve and blindsided. All her worse fears rise to the surface, and she starts to worry about drugs and other concert pandemonium.

At this point, many parents would text their teen, letting him know that the ruse is up and "get home now!" This would be an appropriate response, unless it devolved into a series of emotional exchanges. Stella, however, decides that she could steal her own thunder with a hastily executed text, plus Chris would never open up to her while he's with friends. With a heads-up on his predicament, Chris would have the drive back home to prepare his defense. Instead, Stella phones her husband for his read on the situation. They figure that if Chris were younger and in the middle of a riskier situation, they'd move to extract him immediately. Waiting for him to return will allow for a more focused discussion with Chris about his dishonesty.

By the time Chris walks in the door the next day, Stella has a clear sense of her purpose: to learn the reasons why her usually reliable son would betray her trust. She is ready not only to respond, but to listen as well.

Content *(what is said)*	Process *(underlying dynamics)*
Chris: Hi, Mom! Boy, I'm tired — we didn't get much sleep at Jason's last night.	*Chris wants a cover for his fatigue and a reason for dashing through the hall to his room.*

Content *(what is said)*	Process *(underlying dynamics)*
Chris: Hi, Mom! Boy, I'm tired — we didn't get much sleep at Jason's last night.	*Chris wants a cover for his fatigue and a reason for dashing through the hall to his room.*
Mom (Stella): Hold on, Chris … don't dig yourself any deeper with more fibs. I know you went to the concert.	*Stella knows that she needs to come clean with what she knows in order to get the same from Chris. Nothing is gained by seeing how far he would take the lies.*
Chris: How did you find out?	*After a bust, it's natural for someone to inquire about evidence.*
Mom: Jason's mother told me. Chris — please just tell me what happened.	*As much as Stella wants to express her anger and distress, she knows that unless she stays calm and unemotional, she'll blow her chances for opening up communication channels.*
Chris: You already know what happened. I went to the concert without your permission — obviously.	*Answering his mom with a cynical dig is an effort to be nasty to Mom for busting him and start a fight in order to forestall the vulnerability of confessing his guilt.*
Mom: Chris, I meant the real story behind why you deceived us. It's not like you to do this kind of thing.	*Stella side-steps a potential fight about bad attitude and disrespect, which could easily have resulted in Chris retreating to his room. Instead, she defuses his defensiveness by referring to his usual "goodness" rather than his current bad act.*
Chris: My favorite bands were there, and I knew you'd never let me go. Everybody else's parents were cool with it.	*The best defense is often thought to be a good offense. Chris maintains he had to lie because his parents are deficient and not cool.*

Content *(what is said)*

Process *(underlying dynamics)*

Mom: Families are entitled to their own rules, but that doesn't change the fact that you lied. Why didn't we talk about this? Why didn't you ask permission?

Stella shows remarkable control to ignore the personal slight and stay on focus to gain information and insight.

Chris: Why should I ask? I knew the answer! I knew you'd say no! You and Dad didn't let me go to the state basketball tournament with Casey. You'd just lecture me about safety again!

The dike holding back Chris's anger and resentment breaks.

Mom: Look, that was a five-hour drive over the mountains in the winter. I stand by that decision. But ... oh, Chris ... I had no idea how angry you were about that ... so much so that you'd sacrifice our trust and pull something like this.

It's natural for Stella to feel defensive and "remind" Chris how reasonable her judgment call had been. Nonetheless, she readily and sincerely acknowledges his anger and returns to the focus on trust.

Chris: What trust is there to sacrifice? How much trust are you putting in ME when you treat me like a 12-year-old? I didn't WANT to lie ... but I just figured, "Why play by their rules? There's no payoff. I don't get to do anything."

Chris demonstrates the convoluted moral logic of a kid trying to rationalize his own misdeed by pointing out how his parents sinned first (even more!), making him less guilty somehow for his infraction.

Mom: Hmmm . . . you felt so discouraged by our restrictions that you were willing to take this risk and violate our trust? You felt like we didn't understand your need for more independence?

Stella resists the temptation to defend against Chris' exaggerations and accusations. Instead, she prioritizes listening and empathy — things that aggrieved and angry people want, but rarely get. Stella has a boundary between herself and her son's attacks. This

Content *(what is said)*	Process *(underlying dynamics)*
	allows her to think clearly about her goal of showing Chris she understands his perspective.
Chris: Yeah. That's it.	*By clearly being heard, Chris is relieved and calms down. He's in a position to agree with his mother.*
Mom: I see your point. The thing is, this crisis doesn't exactly motivate me to grant you more freedom.	*Having successfully given Chris space to express his perspective, Stella feels it's time to convey her own.*
Chris: What do you mean? What are you going to do now?	*Chris knows his mom well enough to foresee consequences for his serious violation of trust.*
Mom: Look, Chris, what you did was completely unacceptable. Obviously you'll be grounded. After you've re-established your good record for honesty and trustworthiness, we'll all discuss what new freedoms you feel you need and deserve.	*Now that emotions have settled, Stella calculates that Chris can handle some of the bad news: discipline and reparation for his serious breach of trust. She manages to convey a cooperative plan: Chris needs to establish a better track record and then his parents can try to accommodate more of his perceived needs.*
Chris: How long are you going to ground me?	*Of course Chris wants to know how bad his bad news is.*
Mom: Dad and I will decide together. But Chris … there's one more thing. Please try to communicate your needs directly to us. Going through the back door and lying to get what you	*Stella realizes that this crisis has two parts: the issues of mutual trust and effective communication. Chris needs to express his feelings about his need for new freedoms, while his parents need to realize*

Content *(what is said)*	Process *(underlying dynamics)*
want will never work ultimately. Work with us and then we are beholden to work with you. But you need to talk to us so that we know what you are feeling.	*that if Chris has demonstrated trustworthiness he deserves more independence, even if they are a bit uncomfortable at times.*

Stellar Strategies for Confronting a Teen

This difficult conversation between Chris and Stella proceeded well because Stella kept her head, avoided myriad verbal booby traps and had a more compelling purpose than just punishing Chris. She demonstrated several calm strategies in communicating with her teen in a crisis.

Don't respond to negativity and heat-of-the-moment exaggerations. Most parents would find it irresistible to defend against twisted claims and criticism like those Chris hurled at his mom. Imagine being essentially told, "You made me lie because you were an unreasonable parent." Stella used extraordinary self-control to resist going after Chris' extreme statements, realizing that most people (not just teens) will distort or exaggerate when they are very emotionally upset. **Benefits:** The situation didn't deteriorate. Stella was able hear Chris out and stay focused on getting to the bottom of his dishonesty.

Go with the good. Angry though Stella was, she didn't let her late-night-crisis mentality drive her response. Cooling down and conferring with a spouse helped, but even more importantly, she drew on the deep relationship developed over the years with her son and responded to who he is in the big picture: a basically good kid who pushed his limits and did the wrong thing. Stella didn't mince words. She stayed firm, yet Chris never felt lambasted and put on a guilt trip. **Benefits:** Stella's empathetic manner communicated to Chris that he could trust her to understand his perspective. Discovering that his reasons were symptomatic of a deeper issue, she gained the information she needed to find a more meaningful remedy to his betrayal of trust.

Listen, consider, and mediate the best direction. Parents sometimes sail along thinking all is well until a teen's behavior delivers a jolt. Stella and her husband were operating within their zone of comfort, saying "no" again and again to Chris, who felt that their firmness was unjust. By listening to

Chris, Stella realized she and her husband needed to be more sensitive to Chris' readiness to stretch toward new freedoms. **Benefit:** Everyone learned something, and everyone stands to gain. Chris learned a valuable lesson about honesty and being more up front with his parents. Stella and her husband (who will need to have his own talk with Chris to show him Dad and Mom are on the same page) will set up the discipline so that Chris can re-establish himself as reliable and trustworthy in their eyes. Once his parents regain confidence in him, Chris will be in the position to negotiate for more freedom.

The big benefit: a closer relationship. Much was accomplished in this family crisis because the parents didn't get locked into focusing solely on the "bad" thing their son did. Profound insights can emerge in these kinds of situations. If handled well, a crisis can ultimately bring parents and their teens closer.

Stella didn't let Chris off the hook by any means, but she showed her colors as a good parent by offering him understanding and treating him respectfully, at a time when he expected her to be infuriated. Chris will be all the more appreciative and loving of his parents because they didn't lambaste him for his wrongdoing. He will see them as credible and approachable, and will feel less need to lie in the future. These dynamics build extraordinary intimacy and stronger relationships, which can fortify families for the next adolescent challenge.

Why Even Good Teens Lie

Parents can go into a tailspin over the immorality of lying and react without digging deeper into its origin, function, and motivation. Authoritarian parents are particularly prone to shutting down communication, believing teens need to "learn their lesson" through punishment. Certainly, parents don't want to sanction lying, for honesty is one of the virtues we want our children to take into adulthood. Nonetheless, teenagers will occasionally lie to get what they want or to avoid trouble, and they can still grow up to be honest, especially if they have parents who are truly honest themselves and who work with their child when a lie is detected.

Some families have developed patterns that hinder honesty. Children who are routinely shamed are more prone to lying. Having internalized a fair amount of shame and contempt for their errors, they lack the self-worth to see themselves as good kids. Unable to accept themselves, they wall off their "bad sides" with defense mechanisms such as repression, suppression, denial, and avoidance. Likewise, when parents themselves lie, it breeds a secretive, chaotic family life in which dishonesty doesn't matter and a multitude of poor coping skills become instilled in the children, such as chronic lying to avoid getting into trouble. Families with deep-seated problems such as these should consider counseling, because they will need help beyond the techniques recommended here.

How, then, should parents confront an adolescent who has lied? First, they should present everything they know up front, rather than entrapping the teen with contrived inquiries to see whether he or she will try to cover up. When a teenager lies, address it directly. We could talk about the temptation to lie and how everyone sometimes struggles with the truth. We could discuss how lying can temporarily get us out of a jam, but then we have to pay the cost of our conscience. We might point out how lying contaminates trust between people and how a code of honesty benefits everyone. We can let our children know we'll support their efforts to value truth, even if it means they end up in a jam of another kind. While these exchanges border on the type of moralizing that teenagers inherently turn off, our sincere acknowledgment that lying is a common human foible and that they aren't alone with their dilemma usually keeps their attention.

We don't want to mince words. We can tell them, "You did a terrible thing by lying. We've got to figure out where this deceit is coming from and how you're going to overcome this impulse next time." The point to convey is that lying injures honor and credibility, but they can restore these strengths by prioritizing honesty in the future. We're like cheerleaders encouraging our children. The message to send is "I believe in you! You can do it!"

Setting Up Family Rules and Policies: Don't Forget to Have Them!

Teens sometimes behave as if their parents are a ball and chain around their ankle. Straining for more independence, they can become indignant when quizzed about their plans. "None of my other friends has to tell their parents where they're going" is the classic adolescent line, calculated to make parents feel like freaks for asking.

On the contrary, it's very much the business of parents to stay informed of a teen's whereabouts. Parents are entitled to five questions. The big five are:

- Where are you going? (Include an agreement to be informed if plans change.)
- Who are you going with?
- How will you get there and back? (All transportation information is to be included.)

- When will you be home? (Include a reminder of curfew, if appropriate.)
- What is the contact agreement? (Cell numbers of friends and their parents; promise to pick up/call back immediately if parent calls or texts, with consequences for not responding.)

Remain unflappable, unambivalent, and in lock-step with your spouse (even with an ex-spouse, if possible) about expecting answers to these questions, because parents have a legitimate right to this information. It can help to muster some good humor. If your teen complains, "Why do you always need to know where I am? Don't you trust me?" you can explain that trust isn't all or nothing. Trust is a star we steer by, not an absolute condition. Try saying something like: "I trust you to be a normal teen who may make some moves I don't approve of. I'm narrowing down those possibilities by insisting that you give me honest answers to these five questions." Parents will still need to listen and stretch in other areas, but the big five can serve as their "non-negotiables." As with all family agreements, violations should carry consequences.

Knowing your teen's whereabouts is a starting place for all families of teens. Since shenanigans can still happen, families will need additional rules and policies. Unlike the universal big five, other rules will vary, depending on the needs of the teen and the values of the family. Families should devise policies to govern issues such as curfews, modes of transportation, who is allowed in the home when parents are away, places where teens may or may not go, and types of events they can attend.

The important thing is not to let policies slide, because most teens will find ways to push their limits, often into unsafe territory. Although teens usually want answers "right now," few decisions are as urgent as teens make them out to be. It's fine to explain, "I haven't had time to think this through, but this decision is very much on my mind, and I'll have a response by [a set time, not too far in the future]." A useful policy and rejoinder for parents suffering from teen badgering is "You know the rule. If you keep pestering me for an answer this minute, the answer is 'no.'"

To pin down their specific policies, families can engage in a multistep process. Let's say, for example, that you're trying to determine a reasonable curfew for your 16-year-old daughter. You are the mom, and you feel comfortable with 11 p.m., but your daughter is begging for midnight, and your spouse is leaning toward the later time. Since this is a policy that is potentially negotiable, you can engage in the following four steps:

Do some initial legwork.
- Connect with a few parents whose judgment you trust. Discussing it with others can help you crystallize your ideas. ("I like the fact that family X makes exceptions for big events, but keeps the curfew relatively early for most nights.")
- Try not to make your decisions in a vacuum, but stick with your values. ("I see the advantage of offering a flexible curfew, but I'm not personally comfortable with that. I may be out of line with other parents, but I'm willing to make an effort to enforce my values, even though my daughter will balk.")
- Gather information about how your teenager is handling freedoms in other areas of her life—with school, extracurricular activities, family responsibilities—so you have a larger picture of your child's competence and maturity level. What kinds of situations has she mastered? What needs do you see? Is this a time to pull in the reins or let them out?
- Think back on what your parents might have done and make sure you are neither reacting to their errors nor passing along a parenting style you don't want to sustain. ("My parents were always so strict, so . . . ")

Hold a parent "summit" meeting.
- Share your thoughts and merge perspectives with your spouse so you can act as a united front. Divorced parents can confer with a former spouse or not; different rules in different households can also work.
- Keep in mind that policies are about competency, developed progressively. Children wade, they dog-paddle, then they swim, learning one stroke at a time. Policies should start in a place that allows for growth.
- Teenagers become competent when parents stretch, sometimes uncomfortably so, allowing for trial and error and the development of good judgment. A parallel process occurs: Teenagers learn self-control only when parents gradually relinquish control.
- Consider the worst possible consequence this freedom might carry with it. Is it a potentially lethal issue—one involving cars, for example? The more dangerous the freedom, the more cautiously parents should proceed.
- Whenever possible, try to incorporate the teenager's input and preferences into the policy. This initiates a pattern of responsive parenting, creates an incentive for teens to participate in negotiation, and builds a trust that parents can listen.

Discuss the policy with your teenager.

- Describe to your teenager how you came to your decision, so she'll realize you're not being arbitrary and have thought matters through. If you're sure your newly determined policy is not negotiable, make that clear from the beginning.
- Keep one ear (not both) open to your adolescent's point of view. Although it is in her best interest to push for the outer limit, she may have a compelling case to make.
- As you weigh your daughter's ideas, remember that a parent's comfort zone is not identical to the teenager's. Typically, when parents are completely content with the policy, teenagers aren't. (Just because you want to go to bed at 11, doesn't mean your teenager does!)
- Don't expect a teen to be happy about rules she believes are too strict. Be prepared to handle her indignation. (Only in a bad sit-com would a daughter say, "Mom and Dad, you're right, my Saturday-night curfew should be an hour earlier than everyone else's because I might be too fatigued on Sunday to do an adequate job on my homework.")
- If possible, reassure your teen that if she masters one level, you'll consider moving toward the freedom she feels she deserves. Reward competency by augmenting privilege. This puts tension on the teenager to be responsible, and tension on the parent to loosen the reins. ("If you come in at 11:15 for six months, and all goes smoothly, we'll stretch to midnight.")

Plan a follow-up meeting. Depending on the discussion with the teen, parents can reconvene to process what happened. They may also agree to renegotiate with the teen or make any adjustments to the family rule at a later date.

While determining policies, keep these points in mind: Steady, thoughtful, authoritative parenting can ward off all kinds of adverse adolescent experience. Despite protest, teenagers are often relieved to have rules—when they are fair and consistent. In a pinch, they can call upon their parents' authority or a family policy to save face. Nevertheless, when teenagers believe their parents' policies are too restrictive, they will find ways to maneuver around them. Teenagers seek the lowest denominator of control: If your daughter's curfew is 11 p.m. and her best friend's is 1 a.m., she might seek permission to spend the night with that friend—often.

Using the CALM Technique
Despite parents' valiant efforts and well-devised policies, teens will some-

times pull fast ones on them. Teens' larks will be misguided. They will make huge errors in judgment. And on occasion, they will be defiant, obnoxious, lazy, messy, and unappreciative. Becoming infuriated with a teen is only too easy, but it's an ineffective way to parent.

Unmitigated anger is one of our most disabling emotions. Understanding some of the physiology of emotionality explains why. Whether in conflict or distress, when intense emotions are unleashed, "flooding" occurs. During this aroused state, the heart rate rises, and a release of stress hormones can result in flushing, sweating, and elevated blood pressure. This kind of emotional flooding makes a productive discussion practically impossible. When people are extremely riled up, they experience "cognitive narrowing" into black-and-white thinking, where one's perspective flips into victim/villain, right/wrong, good/bad. Narrowing can lead us to convoluted thoughts like "I'm so angry that you yelled at me. I feel victimized, wronged, and completely innocent, even though I'm yelling, too—in self-defense." Often, both parties feel this way and compete for who is most wronged, and the shouting spins out of control.

What's happening is that with anger and distress, brain activity shifts from the frontal lobes—the center for complex activities such as systematic thinking, achieving perspective, solving problems, and understanding consequences—to the emotional centers of the brain, which include the amygdala, the old, "reptilian" part of the brain.

Our old brains prompt a "fight or flight" reaction, which was useful for prehistoric cave dwellers, but is often maladaptive in our culture, unless we need to escape danger, for example. Angry though we may be, we don't want to cuss out a boss when she promotes someone else, and we don't want to call our kids names and lose credibility. There's truth in the lines of the old song "You always hurt the one you love," because we are less inhibited with our intimate family members and more inclined to let extreme feelings rip. When our reptilian brain has a grip on us, we make distorted, cruel, blaming, threatening, exaggerated statements that never enhance relationships or help discussions.

No wonder parent-teen battles can be so volatile. Immature and still under construction, the teen brain reacts emotionally to practically anything, and when upset, parents likewise fall "under the influence" of their own flooding and reactive emotions. When emotions of teen and parent mix, it's like pouring gas on a fire, now leaping in both directions.

In the midst of strong upset, getting a grip is never easy, but the CALM technique can help you change the trajectory of a heated exchange.

Here is the technique. Say the word "CALM" to yourself and follow these steps:

C—Cool down (self-soothe; control yourself—without trying to control anyone else).

A—Assess options (what are the issues? Would it be better to keep talking or postpone?).

L—Listen with empathy (without any "buts," and when you re-engage, start over).

M—Make a plan (consider ways to handle the meltdown and move forward).

The simple act of going through this protocol and repeating the word CALM may help you shift away from a state of aroused emotions and into a thinking mode.

Here are some more specific principles of good engagement when dealing with difficult, potentially explosive issues. Use them to guide how you communicate with your teen (and others), and to keep highly charged emotions in check.

Stay away from negative openers. Even when grievances are legitimate, starting off with accusations and attacks usually gets people's backs up and leads to angry exchanges. When you want something from someone, stand back from your complaint and think of the best way to package it for "hear-ability" and for inspiring change. Good openers often start with an acknowledgement of the other's perspective, followed by a statement of a desire with an "I" statement. An example would be "I'm sorry we had that argument. I'm sure my concerns about your idea sounded like criticism. Let's figure out a way to negotiate."

Avoid classic negative communication approaches. Included in this list are broad-stroke criticism, globalization ("always," "never"), sarcasm, cynicism, perfectionistic demands, pessimistic forecasting of the future, catastrophizing, ridiculing, belittling, threats, defensiveness, naysaying ("yes, but . . ."), and stonewalling. These tactics hamper problem solving, damage relationships, and diminish trust.

Suggest a cooling-off period if emotions are escalating and you or your teen are in a state of high arousal. A good statement would be: "I feel like I need a 10-minute break to cool down, so I can bring my best efforts to this discussion." Key in this statement is the "I" part, so the other party does not feel abandoned, criticized, blamed, or controlled by the decision for a time-out.

During the time-out, refrain from thinking about your own resentment and indignation, because this will keep you angry and aroused. Instead, try to self-soothe, calm down, and gain a more complex understanding of the problem. Remind yourself that people are different, with varying perspectives, tastes, and preferences. Consider how you might negotiate and what you need to say to be respectful and inspire cooperation. A technique called "paced respiration" can help slow the heart rate down and clear your mind. Using a clock with a second hand, breathe in for five seconds, then out for five seconds, concentrating on and repeating this process until you feel yourself relaxing.

Get back together for a resolution of some kind. Even if it is only to acknowledge regrets and poor communication, work toward an apology and set a mutually agreed-upon date to reconvene.

Be the parent, not the child. In a parent-child conflict, parents are always expected to be more mature, more aware of the need to disengage, and more apologetic if the conflict gets nasty. If a parent tries to take a break (using a statement like the one given above), but the child continues saying horrible things, there is no valid excuse for the parent to keep it up. Responding reinforces the conflict, keeps everyone engaged, and defeats any peace-making process. Disciplining a child for bad language or awful statements uttered in the midst of a battle that the parent has helped to escalate is inappropriate.

To stop an escalating conflict, simply stop talking, even if it means giving the teen the last word.

Consider writing a note or sending a text. Writing allows us to choose our language carefully, stay with "I" statements and be generous to the other party with positive affirmations, particularly after a cool-down period. A heartfelt, polite written expression can be a great way to rebuild a relationship after a destructive, angry outburst. Even if a text is long, teens are likely to read it. They may delete it, but if it strikes a warm chord, they may even archive it.

Remember that short is sweet. The best way to resolve a conflict is to be succinct, acknowledge each other's most reasonable position, and affirm some common ground and interests. Avoid "kitchen-sinking," that is, reviewing every sin, misdeed, and past disgruntlement. Instead, keep the discussion to the core issue and, again, pick your battles.

Let sweet be sweet. Research has shown that the best relationships are those wherein the majority of interactions and verbalizations are positive. To resolve an angry exchange, make an effort to acknowledge whatever reasonable perspective the other party has. Apologies are good medicine to heal wounds.

Dealing With Doubts: Do My Teen and I Have a Good Relationship?

During a big brouhaha, parents can become unnerved, allowing doubts to creep in about their parenting and the whole history with their child. For reassurance, parents need some way to gauge whether their parenting is on the right course and their teen will turn out fine in the end, despite the turmoil. One measure is called "secure attachment." Teens can be way out there in their behaviors, but if they're strongly attached to their parents, there's hope on the horizon.

Secure attachment is defined as the bond children feel to their parents. Growing up, these children feel secure because they perceive their parents to be dependable, trustworthy, and stronger and wiser than they are. For teens, secure attachment will be related to:

- how well attuned and responsive to their needs their parents were during infancy and early childhood
- how parents responded to them when they were upset
- whether they have felt rejected or threatened by their parents
- how they feel their parents have affected their lives and their development

Secure attachment happens when parents are available and emotionally connected to their children. There is a shared awareness in these families that relationships are important and care for others is a priority. Trust and communication are key ingredients.

During adolescence, secure attachment becomes more internally based and is less about actual time spent with parents. Compared to early childhood, teens and parents move toward a more collaborative relationship that allows for more teen autonomy and exploration. Parents continue to be warm and psychologically available; they listen, accept individuality, and are open to some negotiation on rules and responsibilities.

Secure attachment is associated with a raft of highly desirable outcomes, including social competency, flexibility, self-reliance, and curiosity.[1] By late adolescence (end of high school), securely attached teens will tend to agree with these statements:
- My parents respect my feelings.
- My parents accept me for the way I am.
- My parents are reliable sources of support for me.
- I value my parents' perspectives on issues.
- My parents value my opinions on issues.
- When I'm upset, my parents show concern.

If the proverbial fairy godmother appeared and asked for your wish list for your relationship with your child, this would be an ideal list. Of all the things parents hope to give their children, secure attachment is the most enduring positive legacy. How parents handle themselves day in and day out shapes the parent-child attachment, but even more telling is the capacity to weather the storm with grace.

A crisis with a teen becomes a moment of truth in the relationship. When teens have engaged in a prank or other mischief-making, parents feel supremely challenged, but when the crisis involves deliberate deceit, parents feel all the more devastated and disoriented by the personal nature of the breach of trust. To make matters worse, teens often try to wiggle out of trouble, resorting to all manner of distracting illogic to justify their behavior. With flak like this flying in all directions, parents need to steady themselves, assess the big picture of what they want to accomplish, and respond to the "good kid" inside the "bad deed," without letting him off the hook. Instead of just reacting to the wrongdoing with punishment, skilled parents listen carefully and lead the teen to a place where he can face up to his wrongdoing. It takes enormous emotional control—and sometimes anger-management methods like the CALM technique—not to let our reptilian brains get the better of us when teens are pushing our buttons. But when we are successful, a problem becomes an opportunity for growth and learning.

Difficulties with teens can shake parents to their core, create misgivings, and cause parents to wonder if they've failed in their parenting. Remember that almost all families have tough times with teens, and the goals are to manage the problem well, enhance learning, and perhaps even bolster the parent-child relationship in the process. Parents can continue to nurture their teens' secure attachment and internal sense of security when they come through for them. There are no guarantees that everything will turn out OK in a parenting crisis, but a strong bond forged over the years through responsive parenting is the ballast that keeps families steady during rough times.

CHAPTER 4

When You and Your Spouse Disagree

The Family Fish Bowl

On a beautiful weekend, a dad closes his laptop and rallies the family to head outside and enjoy the day. So contagious is his spontaneity that others chime in with suggestions for an outing. With the momentum rolling, family members make each other more creative. The whole mood elevates, generating good energy. A common dynamic, this type of positive snowballing occurs not only in families but in all types of groups.

Our responsiveness to other humans harks back to our core nature as social animals. Now that imaging techniques have allowed researchers to observe the brain in action, we know there's a neurological aspect of people reacting to one another. New research on "mirror neurons" shows that as socially intelligent creatures, our brains are wired to register others' emotions, positive and negative. Someone grins at us, and we're likely to return the grin, not always consciously.

When we walk into a situation, we literally catch the vibe. Consider, for example, how readily a stressful crowd situation, such as a canceled airline flight during the holidays, can deteriorate. With everyone's antennae up, people pick up on the negative and often behave worse in a group than they would on their own. Brain imaging has provided a whole new appreciation for the impact of a loving smile by a parent, and, conversely, for the cumulative effects of constant yelling and shouting in a family, as children's brains register the anger.

Negative snowballing in families can be set off in a split second by an innocuous situation. Consider this example: Stuck in terrible traffic, a mom arrives home in a tizzy and trips over a grimy soccer bag in the entry hall. Loaded for bear because of her bad mood, she expresses irritation over the hallway clutter, complaining globally that "no one ever picks up after themselves." Dad, however, is feeling upbeat because he has spent the last half-hour hearing about his son's exciting soccer match.

In a different mood, he's unable to sympathize with Mom's upset and says, "Chill out. He's had a great game. He came home exhausted and needed to eat something."

Mom feels put down. "Look, we have family rules about dropping stuff in the entryway. Why didn't you make him put his bag away, instead of leaving it to me?" Mom's reaction seems overblown to Dad, and he retorts, "Can't you come home in a better mood? It's no big deal." They're off and running, feeding off of one another's responses.

An inescapable aspect of family life, parents and children ping off each other in myriad ways. In the family fish bowl, one person swerves, and others are stirred by the currents. Even a small movement can set various swooping, diving, or dodging dynamics in motion.

A school of psychology called "systems theory" has been built around this phenomenon to describe the effects of individuals interacting in a group. Family systems theory delves into the ways that family members react to one another, unearthing how and why patterns become established. To understand what's going on with an individual, the larger network of relationships of which he or she is a part is explored. When problems arise in the family "ecosystem," everyone is affected or involved in some way, and everyone can be part of the solution—or not.

Ideally, in a couple's relationship, positions remain somewhat in flux. Sometimes Mom is stressed out and overreacts, but other times, it's Dad. Over time, Mom and Dad complement one another's occasional excesses to achieve balance. But when roles become carved out, and families get stuck in patterns, watch out. If Mom is always the heavy, and Dad always goes with the flow, they are splitting into roles known as "good cop/bad cop."

Some mild version of this dynamic is extremely common in families. At its best, good cop/bad cop can be a conscious family trade. Say, for example, a mom becomes aware of a daughter's sneaking out of the house, but they have been butting heads of late. To keep the relationship from tilting to the negative, Mom can ask Dad—who currently has a store of good feelings with his daughter—to take the lead with this problem. Parents stand together in disciplinary action, but a strategy like this allows each to maintain a mostly positive relationship with the daughter.

The process whereby people become bogged down in extreme, ingrained positions is called polarization. In this detrimental dance, polarization (or "splitting") happens when the exchange of intense emotions drives individuals into increasingly more extreme reactions. Polarization results from a natural impulse to leaven someone else's strong position as we perceive it. When Dad says to his teen, "You can't possible go out the door wearing THAT!" it's tempting for Mom to say, "Oh, that's just the fashion." He's probably too critical, while she's probably too lenient.

In the process of trying to balance out a position perceived as too far out, we rarely express a middle position, instead heading in the opposite direction with a stance that is likewise extreme. One person maximizes, and the other minimizes. As transparent as this process seems, few recognize it in the midst of a quarrel.

Adolescents can ignite polarization between parents. Most teens are risk takers, surging for independence, and because of the vulnerabilities of their brain development, they can lack impulse control and make poor judgments. Teen havoc upsets parents and makes them more anxious. Anxiety, in turn, exaggerates whatever tendencies parents have—for example, toward micromanaging, avoiding conflict, or expressing worries—making it more likely that a spouse will polarize in reaction to the exaggerated trait. In this way, anxiety diminishes possibilities for effective parenting right when you need it most.

Although good cop/bad cop is, arguably, the most common pattern, other polarized positions are plentiful. Each end of the pole has seeds of wrong-headedness and seeds of merit and wisdom. It's the polarization—the process that pushes parents away from a middle position—that's dysfunctional. The solution for each example below is for parents to recognize the problematic pattern and take decisive, cool-headed steps to work toward the middle.

- **The optimist reacts to the pessimist.** A ninth-grade daughter comes home with a midterm grade of C- in math. Dad works himself into a state about it: "I told you we should have disciplined her more about the amount of time she watches TV. She'll never get into college." With Dad forecasting doom and gloom over the C-, Mom is inclined to lighten up. "She's a great kid. It's just a midterm grade, and she's only in ninth grade. Sometimes it takes girls longer to do well in math, and we don't want to discourage her." Pessimism begets optimism, and each parent ends up out on a limb.

- **The "helicopter parent" reacts to the "laissez-faire parent."** An invitation to an eighth-grade party arrives. Dad is inclined to let his son go, no questions asked, trusting his son until proven otherwise, particularly since he's never done much wrong. Mom, on the other hand, is all over it. She needs to call other parents to discuss the level of supervision, and she insists on getting the landline number, so she can phone and make sure he's at the party. "Kids can say they're anywhere with cell phones," she reminds Dad. As the debate ensues, Mom becomes more rigid and determines she'll need to drop by the party, while Dad accuses her of going off the deep end with her distrust. Mom and Dad move to opposing sides (constant vigilance versus leaving kids alone to learn from mistakes), and the process has robbed them of a chance to mediate their positions.

- **The "slacker parent" reacts to the "designer parent."** Dad encourages his daughter to start building her résumé in middle school, packing her schedule with activities selected only toward getting her into the best college. His value on high achievement and attention to status make him ambitious for a path that will take the daughter to the top. Mom believes in letting their daughter just hang out after school and enjoy summers off. The downside of overzealous Dad is that he's ignoring his daughter's interests and preferences, but laid-back Mom also errs by leaving her daughter at loose ends. This family is stalemated.

- **The "unfiltered expresser" reacts to the "stonewaller."** It's Mother's Day, and kids being kids, they do nothing—no card, no festivities. Mom goes ballistic: "After all that I do for this family!" She races through every feeling that comes into her head, no holds barred. Dad just sits there. Thinking that she's not getting through, Mom turns up the volume. "Do you have anything you want to say? Do you want to try to salvage the day before I pack my bags?

    "What do you want me to say? I guess we blew it. We get your message," he responds, but he still does nothing. Dad comes off as ungenerous because he fails to put himself out, but he doesn't want to become a bigger target by defending himself. With Mom as riled up as she is, Dad's instincts tell him to lie low. Dad can't help his inclination to avoid strong emotions any more than Mom can help her urge to express them. Two different personality types have pushed each other to exaggerated versions of themselves.

- **"Martyr Mom" reacts to "Disneyland Dad."** Mom leaves a nice dinner and detailed notes on the kitchen counter for everything that needs to happen when she's out for the evening, from feeding the dog to finishing important school assignments. She returns home to discover dinner dishes in the sink and everyone watching TV. "We'll get it later. The playoffs are on and it's a special occasion," Dad says. Miffed, Mom barks at the kids to go to their rooms to do homework and starts washing dishes herself. Out of her resentment of Dad, Mom has turned into a humorless taskmaster and badger, failing to address the dilemma productively.

Martyr Mom and Disneyland Dad can happen in any family where dads are less attuned to the "to do" list, be it due to travel, divorce, workaholism, or just conventional and rigid gender roles (her job is the domestic realm and kids, and his is the money and yardwork). These dads want to pursue affection, have fun with their kids, and escape the "no's" that effective parents will need to mete out regularly. Moms are fully aware of the duties of childrearing—homework, chores, manners, and so on—and receive the onslaught of negativity associated with the hard stuff of parenting. In the trenches, moms can feel very beleaguered and bitter in their taskmaster roles. Seeking some peace and pleasantness, and wanting to dilute moms' negativity, dads also have a legitimate point, but can end up as ace underminers of reasonable expectations for structure.

From the outside, it's easy to see that each of these split positions is too far out, despite inklings of good in each. Instead of reacting to one another, the optimal approach for parents would be to take parts of each, meet halfway, and parent as a united front:

- The optimist and the pessimist figure out what adjustments should be made for the daughter's TV and study habits, keeping an eye on the possibility of extra help with math.
- The helicopter parent and the laissez-faire parent agree on a couple of reasonable oversight policies for their teen's social life, pulling the fence in closer or moving it out, depending on the teen's behavior.
- The designer parent and the slacker parent evaluate the impact of how their teen is spending her time and create some structure, routine, and sense of purpose.
- Disneyland Dad and Martyr Mom forge a plan for sharing the burden, sorting out opportunities for Dad to take a turn at being the taskmaster, and for Mom to be the good-time girl and throw structure out the window on special occasions.

Sometimes, however, couples have gone too far down the opposite ends of the road with the polarization process and need help. A professional consultation can be valuable when:

- You end up, again and again, in the same entrenched positions, regardless of efforts to soften excesses, make compromises, or shift your roles.

- Discussions with your spouse result in serious discord and/or more distancing.
- Your teen's problem is getting worse because you and your spouse cannot negotiate a middle-zone compromise.
- In spite of mild progress to compromise, you still end up in gridlock and are increasingly losing closeness, affection, or your senses of humor.
- Your positions are becoming more extreme and rigid, and you firmly believe that the other parent is just plain wrong.

Entrenched roles and polarized responses can assume a life of their own. When this happens, parents lose flexibility, perspective, and creativity, and negative feelings abound. A family crisis, illustrated by the following story, can be an opportunity to peer into the family fish bowl and see how the actions of family members have an impact on one another.

Family Story: Parents at Their Wit's End

A family in need of professional help, the Winbushes were at loggerheads over their 14-year-old son, Jameel. Setting up the consultation, Diane Winbush minced no words, describing her son as "messy, disrespectful, and a chronic liar." Her husband, Harris, was, she said, "indulgent" of Jameel. Also in the family was a first-year college student, Ashley, characterized by Diane as "perfect."

A big blow-up over Jameel's marginal school performance and truancy prompted the Winbushes to seek advice. Below is a script from an initial consultation with author Laura Kastner.

Content *(what is said)*	Process *(underlying dynamics)*
Mom (Diane): I know that Jameel doesn't want to be here, but he's had a lot of trouble in school lately. He isn't turning his homework in, and they called us in for a conference because he's just had his eighth unexcused absence.	*Mom starts right up with a negative characterization of her son. Although a presentation of problems is the agenda, this opening statement reflects anxiety and a lack of empathy for how her son would feel about this kind of introduction.*
Jameel: That's bull. I'm in class. They just count me absent because	*Jameel is defensive and counters with provocative retorts. By*

Content (what is said)	Process (underlying dynamics)
I'm late. It's not my fault my locker is so far from my classes. Plus, those teachers enjoy marking me late. It's their form of entertainment.	*blaming others and becoming the victim, he deflects attention from the problems his mother has disclosed. An exaggerated attack on the teachers' motives is meant to bait his mother.*
Mom: Oh, Jameel, you know you're loitering in the halls. You don't make an effort to be on time.	*Jameel has successfully baited his mother and steered the dialogue away from problems that make him feel more vulnerable.*
Jameel (with mock shuddering): Right, Mom, I'm loitering, like a bum in the park. That's what you think, of course. I'm also shooting up and pushing drugs. Why not tell the shrink that one, too?	*Jameel displays his remarkable ability to escalate, push Mom back on her heels, and make it almost impossible to make headway toward a constructive conversation. Since mom looked like she was going to itemize all the things wrong with him, this is an effective defensive strategy.*
Mom (to Kastner): See what I deal with? There is absolutely no way to communicate with him. We have a total breakdown in trust. I can't trust him to do his homework, to go to class, to lock the front door, or to even carry on a civil conversation. Sometimes he calls me at the office, and I can't even trust him to pick up when I call back.	*Diane addresses the therapist, hoping to escape from the exchange with Jameel, which he has easily railroaded. In her frustration, she uses extreme and critical statements about Jameel. Remarks like these almost always alienate and worsen a transaction, despite their ostensible function to get down to business.*
Jameel (laughing cynically): Yeah, two hours later you call me back. Why would I answer? You aren't	*Again, Jameel demonstrates his mastery at hurling stuff at his mother that puts her in a defensive*

Content (*what is said*)	Process (*underlying dynamics*)
so responsible yourself, are you?	*position. Challenging her responsibility is sure to hit a nerve, since that is her greatest complaint about him.*
Kastner: Jameel, your mom uses the word "trust" a lot. What does it mean to you when she says that she can't trust you?	*I've seen enough to know how this dance goes. There is no value in letting them go on with it. My goal is to get to the core issue of why Jameel is so hostile toward his mother.*
Jameel: It means I'm a total screw-up. They treat me like I'm scum of the earth.	*Even though Diane's list of Jameel's bad behaviors and lack of trust are valid and understandable, the overall impact of how his parents have handled things has left Jameel feeling that he is treated like scum.*
Mom: But Jameel, that's not true! We are just frustrated with the way you abuse our home, our trust, and our efforts to reach out to you.	*Although Diane means to say that it is not her intention to make Jameel feel like scum, her defensive clarification only seems to underscore Jameel's point of view.*
	Sometimes when someone criticizes you while trying to act nice, it's more maddening than if he or she just threw a direct insult at you.
Kastner: Mr. Winbush, what is your perception of the problem here?	*The mother-son dance has been unfolding without Dad's involvement, and it's time to pull him into the circle.*
Dad (Harris): Well, it's pretty	*Harris wants to play softball here.*

Content *(what is said)*	Process *(underlying dynamics)*
much like she says.	
Kastner: You seem to kind of sit back and let them go at it.	*I want to point out that non-involvement is still playing a significant role in family transactions.*
Dad: Well, that's sort of the way it usually goes. They both get at each other a lot.	*Harris seems to feel like a helpless bystander.*
Kastner: Mrs. Winbush, what's it like for you, with your husband observing like that?	*I speculate that Diane has felt raw and exposed from her tangle with Jameel, so I want to explore Harris' part in it.*
Mom: It drives me crazy! I do all the dirty work attending to all the problems that go on with Jameel, and he sits back like the Buddha, just watching it all.	*Even though Diane is responsible for her own missteps with Jameel, to be all alone grappling with the messes of your teen, and not doing well at that, is really tough on anyone.*
Kastner: What would you like from him?	*The marital tension here is palpable.*
Mom (with exasperation): Well, a little support of course!	*Often when parents say "support," they mean lockstep agreement. This request is probably more complicated than it sounds.*
Dad: Yeah, but whenever I do try to help, you either cut me off at the knees and tell me I'm coming on too strong or tell me somehow I'm doing it wrong.	*Dad explains that he doesn't get involved because he gets criticized. When one parent observes the other in a fight with a teen, it's striking how "wrong" that approach can seem to the parent on the sidelines.*

Content *(what is said)*	Process *(underlying dynamics)*
Mom (to Kastner): It's just that his temper seems out of control sometimes.	*If fathers don't get lots of practice with involved parenting, they don't have as much "training" in modulating their tempers.*
Dad (confronting Diane directly and harshly): Yeah, to you, maybe. But see—either I'm a lazy Buddha or "out of control." It's no win with you.	*Fathers who feel ineffective and criticized often withdraw and give up.*
Jameel: Yeah, Mom. You're all over everybody. The only one who doesn't give you constant heart attacks is prissy, perfect Ashley.	*Jameel enjoys aligning with his father against his mother about her critical nature. He also likes getting a dig in about his "good" sister.*
Mom: She never speaks ill of you. How dare you . . .	*Diane seems to take the bait every time Jameel throws some at her.*
Kastner (interrupting): You were watching your parents pretty closely there, Jameel, before you chimed in to side with your dad. What would happen if you didn't jump in like that?	*Even though Jameel might be enjoying the alliance with Dad (making Mom squirm and having the focus off himself), it usually makes teens uncomfortable to see their parents in marital conflict.*
Jameel: I don't know. I guess we'd get to watch them drive each other crazy, like Mom said.	*When two people are fighting, a third person often feels compelled to interrupt in order to dilute the intensity.*
Kastner (to Jameel): How helpful of you to draw off the fire. It seems like you are pretty good at drawing a lot of fire, what with the school calling your mom about all of your	*Although Jameel causes problems for his family, he also distracts from his parents' marital tensions by being the biggest identified problem in the family.*

Content (*what is said*)	Process (*underlying dynamics*)
absences and incomplete home-work and so on.	
Jameel: Yeah, I guess that's what I'm real good at—drawing fire.	*Although my positive reframing of Jameel's role as the "total screw-up" is oblique, my hope is that Jameel will know that therapy won't just be about how bad he is.*

Good Cop/Bad Cop: Why Nobody Wins

What is striking about the Winbushes' dynamic is that each family member comes across as both sympathetic and wrongheaded. Each individual contributes to this unfortunate family dance, and each suffers in his or her own way. Diane has every reason to be fed up and distrustful of Jameel. What this young man does in one day is tough to take: He neglects his homework, skips classes, lies, and mouths off to avoid assuming responsibility for his actions. Overwhelmed, Diane feels abandoned by Harris, who has increasingly removed himself from the fray. Feeling he can do no right, Harris has given up and headed for the hills.

Everyone feels powerless. Diane is ineffective in helping Jameel be more successful at school; Harris has hit a wall with Diane's nagging. Jameel can't escape the "problem child" role, and "perfect" Ashley can't make up for her parents' marital difficulties and struggles with Jameel. Given the family woes, she feels there's no room to be a kid and explore her own whims. Like all adolescents, she needs a chance to make mistakes.

What they're doing isn't working. As shown in the script above, Diane fails to see the forest for the trees. Brittle, defensive, and keyed up, Diane reinforces Jameel's baiting by responding to all his gibes, losing credibility and clarity of focus. Harris may look better, but his passivity has left Diane alone with some truly serious teen troubles. He's one of those men who have two settings: on or off. When he's "on," he's losing his temper, but when he's "off," he's stonewalling. Diane's excesses stick out more, but Harris, in his avoidance and occasional fireworks, is equally accountable.

The irony of predicaments like the Winbushes' is that everyone has similar goals: Diane and Harris want to be able to trust Jameel to do his homework and be more respectful. Diane is bone-weary of hounding everyone, while Jameel and Harris want nothing more than to get Diane off their backs. As much as she would love to be less responsible, the devil is in the details of how to make that happen.

Although bigger problems in the family system also needed to be addressed, the behavioral fix involved a restructuring. The short version: Diane was excused from the frontline of parenting, and Harris assumed oversight with the school. Every Friday, he was in charge of going online to review the teachers' updates on Jameel. Jameel's weekend privileges and extra computer time were all contingent on how well he met set goals, as determined by Harris. In this way, Harris re-engaged with the family, learning how to handle some of Jameel's messes.

Diane needed to pull back, relinquish control, and spend some low-key, nonjudgmental time with Jameel to rebalance their ratio of negative and positive interactions. It was no easy job for her to hold her tongue, ignore Jameel's retorts, and trust Harris to do things in his own, looser way.

Jameel had an incentive to cooperate because he got what he wanted—less hassle with his mom—and he tolerated his dad's disciplining better, since he and his mom were equally burned out in their feelings toward one another. Everyone had a role, even Ashley, who needed to get over resenting Jameel and be a sister, not another judgmental "parent."

Many kids screw up in high school, but why did things go haywire in the Winbush family? From a systems perspective, Jameel is the lightning rod. Seemingly maladaptive behaviors, like Jameel's conduct, often turn out to have adaptive functions. Acting out keeps the focus on Jameel and "draws off the fire" from his parents' conflicts. Jameel does not consciously create trouble to get clinical attention or involve his father more, but his behavior brought matters to a crux and had this beneficial side effect.

Parents often enter counseling hoping to "fix this kid," but this can't happen without fixing their family system. Down the line, counseling revealed that the Winbushes were contending with a boatload of issues, including disappointment with their careers, midlife malaise, and losing touch with the positive parts of their marriage. Small wonder that these overwhelmed parents became polarized in their struggles with Jameel.

At the end of their rope when they came into counseling, the family nonetheless mobilized the energy to delve into their myriad problems. Swapping roles, Diane and Harris were willing to try something new that made them each uncomfortable. With this kind of commitment, dynamics in the family improved, and though parenting Jameel will never be a piece of cake, his acting out became less of an ordeal.

How Decent Kids Turn Into Problem Kids

Whether it's a bookworm son who unnerves his sport-loving dad or a girly-girl, non-intellectual daughter who's the object of her feminist scholar mom's fretting, a teen who draws excessive worry from parents can turn into a "problem child." The process can start in adolescence when a teen has a hint of something identified by a parent as a problem. This "something" may need to be addressed deftly, but in its initial phases, it's not major. Clueless about what's normal during adolescence, the parent ramps up the criticism, and the downward spiral begins.

Consider, for example, Nora, a teenager with a laid-back temperament, who isn't very social and is content to sit by herself on the couch watching television. She is in stark contrast to her popular sister Jane, a go-getter and excellent athlete like her dad. Burning a lot of stomach acid over Nora, Dad believes that Nora will be happier if she changes. The following feedback loop illustrates the chain reaction that leads to splitting, or polarization, and creates the "problem kid."

Feedback loop: a family system spiral with a difficult teen

Nora and Dad:

Nora stays home from a dance to watch TV again.

This irritates Dad to no end and he's unable to stay positive. He has little empathy for what might be fueling Nora's problem and expresses his frustration with disdain, "Why don't you just go?"

Nora feels devalued, as if something is wrong with her. She invests less in seeking approval and out of resentment becomes more hostile and nonverbal.

Dad becomes angrier, more hopeless, and more hostile, ranting, "You end up feeling bad, like you have no

Nora feels like a loser, and her behavior further deteriorates.

friends, but you don't do anything about it!

Dad and Mom:

Dad describes his feelings to his wife: "We shouldn't let her be a couch potato!"

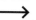

Mom is concerned, but sees Dad's reaction as extreme and harmful. She is aware of harm to Nora's self-esteem if Dad continues to put her down, so she criticizes him for his approach.

Dad resents being criticized for identifying the problem.

Mom identifies with her daughter because she has sometimes been on the receiving end of Dad's critical nature. She knows Nora's actions are part of a bigger problem. She points outs that Nora is not "that bad" and tells Dad he is making it worse.

Dad feels like the bad guy, unsupported by Mom and undermined in his efforts to tackle Nora's problems. This "no win" perception renders him disconnected and he spends more time at work, where he feels more effective.

Mom is caught between her loyalty to her daughter and loyalty to her husband. She's worried about Nora, but worried more about the impact of Dad's negative comments.

How understandable it is for high-energy Dad to be distressed when he sees Nora lounging around at home, outside the social sphere of her peers. But fussing over Nora's behavior spotlights it, to the point that Nora feels belittled and somehow lacking. Reacting to all the negative attention, Nora becomes a victim of her own self-fulfilling prophecy, labeling herself a "loser" who is not good at being social. Having written this narrative for herself, she's more likely to dig herself into a hole. Because of Dad's low threshold of tolerance, Mom becomes Nora's defender. With Mom and Dad polarized, the negative spiral continues downward.

By nature, Nora is a bit of a loner without a lot of fire in her belly. It's just who she is. It's one thing for parents to grind their teeth over their teens' ways in private, but it's entirely another to treat them as if there is something wrong with them. Under the barrage of criticism, teens feel dumped on, and the small problem mushrooms into a big one.

As things stand, Mom is too hands-off with Nora, and Dad is too active. Nora's parents will need to stand together with a compromise plan wherein they insist that Nora sign up for one physical and one social activity of her own choosing. In return, Dad ceases criticism. These activities may not be as much as Dad would like, but they're more than Nora is naturally inclined to do.

The supreme art of parenting is to accept that some characteristics of kids are inborn, and to summon the creativity to manage the teen's behavior—and your own—in a way that keeps the relationship positive and the teen optimistic about herself.

Four Triggers for Splitting Parents Apart

In their worst moments, even the best of parents may slip into polarized positions. Some families, however, are more set up for this process to run rampant. Lives become miserable as bad habits and unproductive roles harden. Splitting occurs for different reasons in different families, and most have a history. Among the most prevalent triggers are the four listed below. Parents who are susceptible to splitting are typically grappling with one or more of these issues:

1. A teen who is harder to parent

Because challenges are intrinsic to adolescence, almost all teens, by virtue of their developmental stage, are harder to parent than when they were younger. Nonetheless, some teens take more work, often because of their temperaments or some diagnosable disorder, such as attention deficit disorder, learning disabilities, anxiety or depression. A classic example of a harder-to-parent

teen would be one who has bad moods, a negative attitude, and angry outbursts. These kids will bite their parents' heads off with little provocation.
Parents can fall into the trap of mostly negative reactions, a sure path to family discord and distress between parents.

Changing the course: Don't blame your child for inborn biology. Fed
up and overwhelmed, parents may have the best of intentions, but they rarely grasp how confused and lost their kids feel. When teens are stirring the
pot—made worse by parental negativity—they invariably see themselves as
the family screw-up. Feeling unappreciated and hopeless, they have little incentive to act better.

Teens with challenging temperaments require better-than-average behavioral management skills. In a nutshell, parents will need to reinforce positive
behaviors, while ignoring many negative ones. They'll need to provide incentives for behaviors they want to develop, while doling out negative consequences in the form of lost privileges for behaviors they want to discourage—all the while maintaining a loving, upbeat relationship. And when there
is a "perfect" sibling receiving all the fairy dust, parents will need to pour on
the love to the more aggravating child, even though it feels unnatural.

It is up to parents to create a boundary and not respond to verbal garbage
from a mouthy, irritable teen. Parents who are aroused and talk too much
lose ground. They may feel that raising their voice establishes power, but it
doesn't. Negative attention is still attention, reinforcing more bad behavior
and defiance.

These parents will encounter many moments where they need to stay calm
and make a conscious choice not to react, returning to an issue at a better time
with a better approach. Seeing the bigger picture and feeling empathy for a
harder-to-parent child takes superhuman insight, given how scared, anxious,
frustrated, and powerless parents can feel.

2. "FOO doo": Family-of-Origin baggage

All of us have something we want or don't want for our teens. Sometimes,
our hopes and expectations relate more to our own pasts—our "family of
origin"—than what's good for our kids. Extreme or distorted expectations
can create conflict and splitting between spouses.

No matter how you fill in the blanks, it's worth some soul searching:
"Because of these things I cherished, I want to re-create _____ for my kid."
Or, "Because of these regretted experiences, I intensely want or don't want
_____ for my kid."

One example might be a parent raised in poverty who showers her teen with material goods to protect her from want. Another classic is the parent who avoids conflict and determines to stick out a miserable marriage, no matter what, because her own parents were divorced.

Also classic are parents who panic when they think they see "the bad family gene" in their teen. For example, if a mom has a "n'er do well" sibling still living off her parents or even with a mental health problem, she may overreact to a normal teen mishap, fearful that her teen is headed in the same direction.

Changing the course: Insight is the first step. Wading in "FOO doo," parents can become blinded to what their child actually needs. With a misguided agenda, it's easy to overlook important realities that should be considered, such as a spouse's values, a teen's capacities, or life circumstances. The result: disagreements on how to parent.

Once family baggage is front and center, parents can begin to identify patterns. If, for example, a mom was wounded by a dominating, insensitive dad and her husband starts to look too commanding, she'll need to guard against comparing the two. Or if a dad struggled in school and his child starts to look scrappy and have conduct issues, he can remember to rein in his reactivity.

3. Ruts in the road: The myth of clear skies and happy trails

How innocently we head into the future, with little awareness of problems that can undo our dreams! Particularly with middle age, stressful circumstances can strike, whether they're health problems, elderly parents, extended-family issues, work stress, financial setbacks, or marital struggles. Major hurdles can sap our ability to stay primarily positive with others, take care of our health (sleep, exercise, nutrition), pick only crucial "battles," and save energy for crafting a good life. The countless challenges of normal marriage, normal teens, and normal life are vastly underrated and can trigger splitting in parents.

Changing the course: Accept the inevitability of life stressors. Bad things can happen, and for significant life traumas, people need support instead of acting in isolation. Sometimes, however, we can crumple too easily under the weight of circumstance, adopt a beleaguered attitude, and lose out on the opportunity to grow through challenges. Whatever the "rut in the road," try to commit to a positive problem-solving approach. Life isn't easy, but flexibility, optimism, and finding what gives you pleasure can ease the way.

As a philosophical position, Reinhold Niebuhr's Serenity Prayer says much. To paraphrase this gem, we should seek the serenity to accept the things we can't change, the courage to change the things we can, and the wisdom to know the difference.

4. Partnership paradoxes: First comes attraction, then comes detraction.

Unresolved marital differences can propel polarization and deprive parents of their resourcefulness. People marry for all sorts of rhyme and reason. One pattern known to marital therapists is marrying to complete yourself, as if two "better halves" would constitute a whole. A quiet, introverted man might, for example, fall for a social butterfly who can make up for his social awkwardness.

Sometimes partnership paradoxes work like a charm. But not always. The trait that initially acts like a magnet and seems desirable in a partner can also be the thing that drives spouses crazy later in marriage. The old saying "Fire in the heart can put smoke in your eyes" speaks to how couples in love see only the good and overlook characteristics that may alienate them over time.

Changing the course: Get the big picture of how marriage works and become aware of your own excesses. Individuals often enter into counseling bent on changing their spouse. Consider asking instead, "What can I do to change myself, so that I'm not reacting?" Typically, this involves shifting perspective to see that the bothersome trait is the underbelly of something good that attracted you to your spouse in the first place. A wife who can't endure her husband's workaholism can appreciate that she fell in love with him because he was an ambitious superachiever. A husband who is irritated because his wife runs the home "like a boot camp" can recall how drawn he was to her competence and strong will.

More likely than not, the insufferable characteristic is an aspect of a trait that was once valued and chosen. Moreover, we all need to have some humility about our own underbellies, addressing our own self-improvement instead of reacting to another's behavior. This kind of big picture can diminish rancor.

Hidden problems in a marriage often result in patterns such as polarization, lack of cooperation, or stonewalling, all of which have an impact on kids' behaviors. Couples who have little interest in marriage counseling will still seek therapy for their children's problems, but during counseling, the debris below the surface rises upward. Out pour all the issues that have been ignored, such as alcohol use, sexual problems, undiagnosed depression, money fights, her intolerable bitchiness and repressed anger, his cold egocentrism and "not getting it."

This sounds like a list of classic problems, but the point is that many parents have marital issues perceived to be "not enough" to bother with therapy. Or they may be afraid of counseling, fearing that it might accentuate problems and threaten marital stability even more. But those problems can end up manifesting themselves in disagreements over the kids, non-collaboration, and inadequate problem solving for the difficult challenges of the teen years.

Compared to the relatively serene waters of earlier years, adolescence will rock the family boat. Only too easily can parents disagree in their assessments and reactions, whether pertaining to a specific incident, such as a teen prank, or a more global issue, such as teen rudeness. Whatever the dilemma may be, no matter how exaggerated, off-base, or just plain wrong a spouse's position seems, a knee-jerk reaction in the opposite direction is always detrimental to the family system.

Splitting robs parents of one of the most valuable assets of any parenting system: two good minds joining forces to solve a problem. With the benefit of one another's combined perspectives, parents will almost always have a fuller view and a more effective united parenting approach.

CHAPTER 5

When Your Teen is Acting Like a Spoiled Brat

The Epidemic of 'Entitle-mania'

Call it "entitle-mania": The average American kid has more stuff, wants more stuff, and gets away with fewer chores around the house than any previous generation. Not limited to the affluent, this trend cuts across all socio-economic classes. As parents, we haven't made it a priority to train our children to roll up their sleeves and fully participate in daily household drudgery. As a result, many kids today feel entitled to all the benefits of family life without giving much back. Teens might work plenty hard in school and have crazy-busy extracurricular schedules on top of that, but family duties aren't a big part of their job description.

This is a pickle we've created. Many parents feel that their teens are spoiled, but degrees of spoiled range from "somewhat" to "excessively." Most teens are in the "somewhat" category: They pout and drag their heels, but ultimately do some chores. Most teens also have healthy appetites for goodies such as clothes, electronics, and athletic gear, spending on average about $112 per week.[1]

Teens being teens, they'll use their verbal and emotional talents to try to persuade parents they *have to have* something and, likewise, to get off the hook with family jobs. Compared to parents previous generations, we place more of a value on our children's feelings than on strict obedience, meaning that kids are freer to express feelings and, fortunately or unfortunately, we are likely to hear them. When we insist that they rake leaves or sweep floors or we deprive them of their wants, we hear their pity party. They tell us we're meaner than other parents, that nobody has it so bad, or the big mud sling: "My friends feel sorry for me."

Although still controversial, another generational change pertains to increased levels of narcissism in teens found in research.[2] With all of the "specialness" conferred on children today, why wouldn't they get the sense that it's "all about me"?

Family Story: A Parent's Plan Backfires

The reality check is that most teens don't do chores with smiles on their faces. Hearing teens whine and complain is one thing, but giving in to it and reinforcing these behaviors is another. Truly indulged teens can become downright defiant about chores; meet Victoria Perkins.

Over the years, Sandy and Bob Perkins took a stab at holding their daughter responsible for some family tasks—emptying the dishwasher, folding laundry, walking the dog—but these expectations invariably fell apart in the face of her many convincing excuses. Often asked to lend a hand, and often threatened, Victoria always had something more pressing to do.

Like many parents, Sandy and Bob knew they should hold her accountable, but their crammed schedules and busy lives outdid their best intentions. Suffering from time famine, the Perkinses didn't want to spend precious family moments breathing down their children's necks. Only too quickly, kids figure out that if they make it really, really hard on their parents, they stand a better chance of getting out of things they don't want to do. Instead of enduring the unpleasantness of enforcing family chores, Sandy and Bob took the path of least resistance and did the jobs themselves.

By the time Victoria finished middle school, her parents had reached a breaking point. They turned to each other and said, "She's 14 and does nothing around here. This has to stop." Going for broke, they decided to hold out a huge carrot: the money needed to attend her eighth-grade graduation party at a waterworks park. Sitting down together with Victoria, they told her she would have to earn the money for this important party by weeding the back yard and sweeping the garage. As the date approached, Victoria wasn't doing it. The more her parents reminded her, the more uppity she became. Everyone was on edge as they headed for a showdown.

Bursting with frustration, Dad brought it up again with all the subtlety of a sledge hammer.

Content *(what is said)*	Process *(underlying dynamics)*
Dad (Bob): You know the deal: If you don't get to those chores we talked about, you won't have the money for your school party.	*Even though Dad intends a mere nudge and reminder that Victoria needs to take their "deal" seriously, he opens with a threat.*
Victoria: Why do I have to work for my graduation party? Everybody else's parents are nice enough to just pay for it.	*When kids know two or three friends with a situation that promotes their case for parental injustice, it becomes "everybody."*
Mom (Sandy): Victoria, we give you an allowance and yet you	*Mom fell for her daughter's exaggerated provocation. Her defense*

Content *(what is said)*	Process *(underlying dynamics)*
don't hold up your end and help out at all around here. We're fed up. We just want you to weed the back garden and sweep out the garage. It's not asking too much.	*that the chores are reasonable is sure to fall upon deaf ears.*
Victoria: Ugh (heavy sigh of disgust)! The garage is a mess, and the garden is a jungle. I can't believe you guys are doing this to me.	*A 14-year-old who has never been expected to do chores is likely to feel like a victim despite her parents' logic that it is high time that she starts helping out.*
Dad: We gave you plenty of time to earn your way, Victoria. You're spoiled rotten and know it. We can't keep bank-rolling your million pleasures without seeing some effort from you.	*Dad is easily triggered because this issue has been brewing for a while and the power struggle is in full gear.*
Victoria: Yeah, well— whatever, Dad (sounding truly indifferent).	*One of the most maddening power plays around is the "blow-off."*
Mom: Victoria, I honestly don't think that a few chores are too much to ask for.	*Victoria has reversed the power dynamic such that Mom is now pleading.*
Victoria: You're making such a big deal about this. Don't worry about it—I'll just borrow the money from Sophie. (She turns on her heel and exits.)	*Since Victoria knows perfectly well that the "deal" was about earning her way to the party and not funds per se, this passive-aggressive move packs quite a punch.*
Dad: You wait just a minute here, young lady. You're not getting away with that crap. We're not about to let you go to that party!	*A counterpunch of this magnitude might be understandable, but it won't result in cooperation, a lesson learned, or character development.*

The Big Brush-Off: A Teen's Favorite Weapon

When chores are incorporated into the family routine, parents are contributing to their child's character development. One of the beacons of childrearing, character development includes instilling a sense of responsibility, an expectation to give back to the community of home, and a work ethic. These behaviors, desired by all parents, are the opposite of "spoiled rotten." Small wonder that Sandy and Bob Perkins went to the mat for them. If, however, parents wind up in a jam, unable to muster any cooperation and faced with significant power struggles and noncompliance, it's a tip-off to rethink the approach.

While it's high time for Victoria to help out, her desperate parents fixated only on that goal, without giving adequate thought to the process. Their eyes were on the right prize, but they took the wrong path.

For starters, the Perkinses committed key missteps in communication. Parents risk instigating power struggles when they:

- Impose a big, empty threat. Threats always raise hackles and put teens (or anyone) on the defensive.
- Commit errors of insults, exaggerations, and "you" accusations, without any affirmations that would inspire a teen to consider going along with the program.
- "Pile on" grievances, dwelling more and more on how parents feel without regard for how the teen feels. Although "empathy" with a bratty teen is difficult to feel, the deal will flop without it.
- Fail to put a halt to the exchange when it's clear from the beginning that there's no collaboration and virtually no chance of motivating a teen with more criticism.

It wasn't just the Perkins' errors in communication that worked against them; their entire plan was ill conceived and bound to fail. Without engaging Victoria in any way, they imposed a heavy-handed dictate with an enormous negative consequence—not going to the graduation party. This proved a serious flaw in the plan; Sandy and Bob didn't really want her to miss out on something as special as this party—and don't think she didn't know this!

Victoria's parents are resentful because she isn't pulling her weight in the family, but how did she become a kid who scoffs at chores? Victoria is a slacker because of all the tough parenting work that her parents didn't do along the way. She is "spoiled" because her parents have been ineffective. Getting kids to do chores takes years of training, starting with toddlers who pick up some of their own toys, progressing to youngsters who clear dinner dishes, and leading to teens who feel obliged (albeit begrudgingly) to participate in household tasks as a matter of course.

Coming in high and mighty, Mom and Dad are starting from zero with a teen who has a history of doing zilch. They're trying to leap too far in one step, and she feels overpowered. Victoria's response to her parents' mandate is standard practice for teens: Faced with a demand that strikes them as unfair and unexpected, they will resort to passive-aggressive behaviors; that is, they will express their defiance, resistance, and opposition by *not* doing something. To get back at their parents, they'll cut off their nose to spite their face.

Ranging in severity and intent, passive-aggressive behaviors could include:
• Acting willing but never getting around to it
• Intentionally completing the task in a poor way
• Whining and wheedling their way out of the task
• Interrupting with distracting, resistive comments and a hostile attitude

A degree of passive-aggressive behavior comes with the territory of adolescence. Every time our teens blow us off, withhold information, or won't talk at the dinner table, there's an element of passive aggression in play. This happens because we make many demands on our kids; we need to be sensitive to how heavy-handed our nagging can be. Anything can become a power struggle when parents are too much "at" their teens, even if it's all for a good cause.

Teens can win a power struggle by the power of "not." They lack the authority to withhold their parents' allowance, ground them, or take their car keys. But maddening passive-aggressive ploys give them the power to drive parents crazy. Failing to stay calm, parents can become unhinged and wind up trying to control too much or too little.

An all-too-common dynamic plays out like this:
Parent: Makes a good call to impose some authority and hold the line with a chore.
Teen response: Pitches a fit and does nothing.
Parent, next move: Fit to be tied, parent nags and nags.
Teen response: Becomes snarky, punishing the parent through obnoxious behavior, while still doing nothing.
Parent's next move could be: Doubting himself, thinking, "Things have gotten too hot. It's not worth it." He folds and feels ineffective.
Result of folding: The teen has succeeded by wheeling her way out of what she sees as a hardship.

Or, parent's next move could be: Holding the line while still suffering from the heat in the relationship and nastiness of teen.

Result of holding the line: Teen experiences negative consequence for not cooperating, but has succeeded by making her parent miserable, too.

The Perkinses have dug themselves into a hole with the near-certain likelihood that everyone will lose. If Dad follows through on his threat, Victoria misses this special party; her parents feel guilty and sad that she's lost out; and the parent-teen relationship will suffer. Nothing good is going to come from sticking with a bad plan. The best move for parents in this situation is to regroup and put an end to the power struggle.

Calmly and respectfully, Victoria's parents can describe the dilemma as they see it, with even a hint of deference that perhaps the original plan wasn't coordinated well. They can maintain their position by insisting that Victoria needs to do something toward the goal of earning money for the party, but they can brainstorm with her to figure out what she is willing to do. It may even be something outside the home, such as baby-sitting for the money. The key is to get her to buy in. In this way, everyone wins: Victoria gets to go, her parents don't feel terrible, the relationship is intact, and Victoria has made one small step in the direction of being more responsible.

The Usual Slog With an Average Teen

Victoria is an extreme example, but today's average teen is sloppy, inconsistent, and reluctant to do chores. This is the norm: Today's teens rarely snap to it.

The more that families make household duties a way of life for kids, the more easily children will comply because they're accustomed to it. Authoritative parents hold the line, tolerate some guff, and build up a history of meaning what they say with reasonable expectations. But even under these circumstances, teens will probably show some attitude, parents might have to ask more than once, siblings might argue over whose turn it is, and there might be some tiffs and theatrics and a hard lesson or two. We may feel like calling them a "spoiled brat," but resistance and self-centeredness are the stuff of the teen years, so it's up to us to stay calm and firm.

Parents should do the best they can, with the goal of keeping nagging and reminding to a minimum. A parent might keep it light, saying something like, "Oh, come on now, you're 15. Don't make me have to discipline you by pulling your allowance." Or a parent could say, "You don't like being badgered, and I don't like your heel dragging. Let's make a deal and figure out when this will be done." Other good tactics include linking privileges—and consequences—to the completion of chores. While parents should expect 100 percent compliance on family responsibilities, they shouldn't expect teens to be pleasant about it, nor should they expect the highest-quality job. Shoddiness and sour pusses are a teen's desperate attempt for some power in the equation.

Q & A: How to Kick-Start New and Better Habits for Truly Resistant Teens

The challenge is far greater when parents have a history of inconsistency with expectations, and teens have become accustomed to receiving something for nothing. If parenting has been sloppy, teen behaviors will reflect that. The following frequently asked questions pertain to situations in which teens are flat out resisting their responsibilities and as a result, parents are nagging, threatening, and ready to blow their tops. These predicaments involve not only doing chores, but situations such as practicing an instrument, doing athletic drills required by a coach, getting up in the morning on schedule, doing homework, or completing extracurricular tasks such as summer reading.

For parents needing to initiate new and better habits for defiant teens, here are common questions:

Q: What's wrong with cutting to the chase and letting kids know exactly where you stand with a "do it or else" statement?

A: Threats and ultimatums are like red flags in front of a bull. They are more likely to arouse defiance and counterattacks than cooperation—especially with an unruly teen. Simply put, these strategies are not as effective as negotiated deals. Whether it pertains to chores, practicing piano, or doing Hebrew lessons, there needs to be an ongoing, working alliance, which rarely results from threats and punishments.

Sometimes, however, parents can be successful in stating their limits, as long as they follow through. Let's say your teen is in the habit of staying in bed too long and missing her carpool. After a couple of reminders, make your position clear: "This is your last chance. Next time, I'm not driving you. You'll need to ride your bike or take a bus." The teen may hate your guts for not driving her when she blows it again, but she'll be getting herself out of bed earlier in the future.

Q: If angry ultimatums don't work, why do parents often wind up using them?

A: Recognize ultimatums as a desperate measure. They slip out of parents' mouths as a result of frustration, when parents have reached the end of their rope. Feeling powerless to get what we want from our kids, we resort to a big threat, hoping that the power of "or else" will give us the upper hand. Power struggles are just that—a struggle for power—and not an invitation to work toward a solution.

Q: *What's wrong with using something teens really want to do—such as going to a party—as leverage? Why not restrict them from going unless they do as we wish?*
A: Once in a while you may have to do this, but a steady stream of negative threats doesn't inspire a good relationship. If we've already consented to something, even tacitly, it's playing dirty pool and being coercive to yank permission at the last minute. To be effective, parents need positive strategies instead of punishments.

Parents can, however, flip the language and set up incentives. Giving the teen plenty of notice, we can say, "When you finish your reading, I'll drive you to the mall."

Q: *What about enticing a teen with something highly desirable and out of the ordinary, such as a special birthday celebration, a car, or a new puppy?*
A: This is almost always a bad idea, because parents as well as teens buy into special things emotionally. Parents then have grave misgivings about withdrawing the offer if the teen isn't successful. Parents should never create situations (promises or threats) they're not willing to follow through on, because to do so erodes their credibility. And they shouldn't shoot for a goal beyond the teen's reach, since it sets the teen up for failure.

Q: *How can parents gauge whether a goal is out of reach?*
A: If the teen hasn't shown any motivation to start the new habit, and may even have expressed a loathing for the task, it is unrealistic to expect that she will all of a sudden flourish—out of the blue, on her own—in that area, no matter what the reward.

Q: *What's the best way to kick-start a new habit or a new regime?*
A: Basically, break it into chunks. First, negotiate the "new program," preferably with input from the teen. Second, supply small rewards for small steps in the right direction, which are easily earned and easily taken away, without a lot of drama. Third, adapt the program as needed, since

we rarely hit it exactly right from the start. A new habit takes time, repetition, and rewards along the way in order for it to take root.

Q: *But why would teens ever agree to do something they really don't want to do—chores, for example?*
A: Tell them straight out that chores are a non-negotiable responsibility. Part of a parent's job is to prepare children for the world, and this is the way of the world: First you do your work, then you get your reward. There are, however, negotiable terms. Teens can be allowed some say on which chores, which deadlines, and which rewards. The difference in attitude can be like night and day, because they buy in to the task through their participation.

Q: *What if the teen is the one proposing a big reward, pleading that this is just the ticket for motivating them?*
A: Teens don't always know what's good for them, since certain kinds of "all or nothing" propositions can put too much at stake. When the big reward is time sensitive (a trip or experience, for example), parents can find themselves in a real bind if they have to yank it. As the deadline nears and the teen's performance is (almost always) hit or miss, everyone's anxiety increases. When teens feel unsuccessful, their anxiety can come out as anger, irritability, and nastiness. With increased tension, relationships suffer. Plus, the teen may have his heart set on this wonderful experience. By not earning it, the bad blood that results in the relationship could last longer than any lesson learned.

If the big reward has no pressing deadline—say, a consumer item like a bike or a laptop—teens can earn points toward the reward over time. Still, the teen has to be motivated and have the staying power to stick with the system.

Q: *Why are small rewards usually better than a big one?*
A: Small rewards allow parents to be comfortable with giving and taking away. For example, for every day's completion of chores, the teen earns the next day's screen time. No completion, no screen. And if the reward stops working, we change it to something else, perhaps a social freedom. With small steps, parents are able to tweak the system along the way and help the teen succeed.

Q: *What if my teen already has everything she could possibly need or want? Does it make sense to heap more rewards on a teen who already has too much?*

A: Therein lies the rub. It's hard to give more goodies to an indulged teen, but rewards work better than punishment. From the teen's perspective, doing the new task is burdensome. Moody teens tend to overestimate the awfulness of the new habit, whether it's studying more, practicing an instrument, or being tutored. That's why we override their resistance with the goody. If necessary, parents may need to revoke privileges previously given, and make these perks contingent on task completion, but they should expect protest.

Q: *Other teens in other families do chores without being rewarded. Why shouldn't my teen take them on as part of being in the family?*
A: Typically, teens who automatically help out have had those patterns up and running from early in their lives. Parents frustrated by their "spoiled kids" are also upset with themselves because they didn't do the chore of establishing chores during middle childhood, when it would have been easier. At this point in the game, forget about the way things should be. The basic question isn't "what's right?" but "what works?" Positive reinforcement works best for reversing bad habits.

Q: *What if we've agreed to a plan and a few weeks in, it's not working and it's clear the teen is going to fail? Should we stick with the program in the interest of being consistent?*
A: Call it off. If the teen isn't going to succeed, there's no reason to keep going. Come up with something else. Consistency is desirable once you have the new routine under way. Good parenting involves consistency and stability, but it also requires adaptability and innovation. In this instance, it's perfectly OK to say to the teen, "Look, what we're doing isn't working. We need to adjust the plan to get back on track."

Q: *What if we thought we had the new habit established and have doled out the rewards, but everyone got busy and, lo and behold, the teen has lapsed and is resisting?*
A: This is where consistency matters. Parents will need to come up with fair and effective consequences for noncompliance. It should be a measure that's easy to impose and within the parent's power, and it should follow a reasonable logic and not be unduly harsh. Basically, it's "You'll get to do X when you've done Y."

Q: *Should consequences for noncompliance be clear from the outset, so teens know what's in store, or is that a threat?*

A: Consequences should be clear, but the program needs to be presented in positive terms. For example, "You finish your chores by 8 p.m. nightly, and you get your cell phone for use the next day." If they don't do it, no hand-off of the cell phone. Emphasize the positive, root for the teens' success, and say little—no threats, no finger wagging—when they fail.

Q: Isn't it unrealistic for parents to stay quiet when teens are throwing a hissy fit about not having something they believe is their due, such as cell phone privileges?

A: The only person we can control is ourselves, and the blow-up will be less intense if we remain composed. Teens will protest, but this is intended to get parents to cave, feel bad, rethink their authoritative stance, or just feel miserable. From a teen's perspective, the new regime is bad news.

Q: What if my teen continues pitching a fit?

A: Things often get worse before they get better. Most indulged kids are very good at wearing parents down. Because tantrums have worked before, teens will not only keep at it, they'll double the intensity—following parents into the bathroom, telling parents they hate them, threatening to go live with Aunt Betty. This is called "extinction surge." Their freak-out is an honest, intense emotion, as if to say, "How dare you change the program on me like this!" The surge is also their last-ditch effort to weaken the parents' resolve. Withstanding their wrath can be dreadful the first time, but behaviors will improve once teens know their parents mean business.

Q: Is it ever just too late and not worth the effort?

A: The later parents take action, the more inconvenient it will be. What's important is to keep your anger out of it. In the same way that brushing teeth is not up for grabs, teens can acquire a habit and be trained to get up from the table and do the dishes. Routine is a beautiful thing. Nonetheless, parents always have to establish priorities and not have too much of an agenda at any one point in time. To preserve a "mostly positive" rapport, many parents simply let go of some of the battles, like always keeping a room clean or staying up late to do homework, saving their effort for more pressing issues.

Q: Most parents give allowances without tying them to chores, but sometimes money is the only way to get a spoiled teen's attention. Is there a point where you draw a tough line at "no chores, no allowance"?

A: Absolutely, but delivery and tone are everything. Start with an apology that you regret you didn't start this program earlier. Make sure you are clear and neutral in tone about how privileges need to be earned, based on the completion of chores and responsibilities, leaving out threats and criticisms. Then stay calm while weathering the storm.

Family Story: If I Say 'Yes,' Will My Teen Love Me More?

Alice Louvack was tied up in knots. No matter how much she did for her son, it was never enough. A committed mother who adores her son and works hard to be a perfect parent, she would plan nice occasions or buy him the latest electronic gadgets. Allen's appreciation would last about five minutes before he was slouching on the couch, bargaining and wheedling for the next thing. Although he also went after his dad, Mom was experiencing more conflict with Allen, and she felt harassed, unappreciated, and taken for granted.

Alice also had problems disciplining Allen. Rules didn't stick. Not a major trouble-maker, Allen caused lots of little headaches by violating curfew, running up online charges, or borrowing valuable family belongings and leaving them at a friend's house. Whenever Alice imposed consequences, Allen would finagle a way around them. Alice realized she had trouble setting limits and recognized her own complicity in spoiling Allen, but she still couldn't make sense of why he was, in her words, "so manipulative."

One late afternoon, Allen pursued his mom again in this way:

Content *(what is said)*	Process *(underlying dynamics)*
Allen: Hey, Mom, we've gotta go to the mall and get those new shoes for the dance tonight. Hurry! We're all meeting at 6 at Jess' house to get ready. C'mon!	*Parents are often put in the position of responding to their kids' urgent demands. Hearts pounding, kids experience their needs as a crisis.*
Mom (Alice): Allen, you can't be serious! There is no way I'm going out in Friday rush-hour traffic. You have other shoes. Plus, I have to get ready for my own plans tonight.	*If only a parent's perspective on apparel options could quell a teen's desperate need for the perfect look!*

When this kind of absorption occurs, emotions are amplified, and the inundated person isn't able to use her thinking brain or choose what to say. By contrast, people with rigid boundaries may "shut down" in emotional situations. Because their boundaries are operating like impenetrable walls, they're unable to take in and appreciate another person's thoughts and feelings. But on occasions when they do absorb emotions, they may feel like they're going to explode.

With healthy interpersonal boundaries, we don't have to tell another person everything we think and feel. We keep our private thoughts to ourselves and decide what is best to share given: 1. the type of relationship (parent? child? stranger? boss?); 2. what we're trying to accomplish (instruction? avoiding hurt? de-escalating conflict? buying time to calm down?); and 3. our sense of the likeliness that a productive exchange can happen if we express our thoughts and feelings (is the person receptive? able to comprehend our point?).

Parents who lack firm interpersonal boundaries with their children leak too many of their own feelings and absorb too many of their child's emotions and attitudes. This type of relationship is often called "enmeshed" or "symbiotic." If the child is riled up and anxious, so, too, is the parent. As the duo becomes increasingly upset, a circular reaction is triggered, which can easily get out of control, destroying warmth, communication, and any chance of judicious decision-making or discipline.

As Alice Louvack quarrels with her son, her boundaries become so blurred that his hostility rushes straight in. Bowled over by his tantrum, Alice regresses into sibling-like bickering with Allen, unable to give him the parenting he needs.

Alice and Allen are "co-flooding." Essentially, Alice is upset that Allen is upset about her "no." Outraged that he is setting her up to be the "mean mommy," Alice's heart rate increases to 90 beats a minute. Allen is frustrated, imagining himself a loser at the party, so his heart rate races to more than 100 beats a minute. Continuing to react to Allen's upset and frustration, Alice becomes even more excitable and panicked, thinking she is trapped into going to the mall, dealing with traffic, and being late to her own event. Saying "no" is not an option for Alice, because her son will hate her temporarily, and she can't tolerate it.

Parents secure in their role can withstand a teen's fury without feeling crushed, keep a good self-image, and create their own script, which could be something like this: *My son will get through this rage and disappointment. I'm a good parent for teaching him that tantrums don't work. To be strong and independent, he has to learn that he can have fun at the dance without new shoes. I'm doing what I need to do, even though this is hard.* In the midst of a fight, a parent can use the CALM technique (Cool down; Assess options; Listen with empathy; Make a plan), take a break and self-soothe with a similar inner dialogue.

Parents who find it impossible to say "no" with conviction often grew up in difficult circumstances, with problems in their families of origin. Weak boundaries can result from any kind of hardship: poverty, trauma, alcoholic parents, domestic violence, family mental illness, neglect, or an insecure relationship with parents. Shaky parenting can result whenever a parent says, "I always wanted to give my child the X I didn't get," with X standing for affection, opportunity, resources, or a smooth life, for example. No matter how many books a parent reads on what one "should" do, until the impact of a difficult background is understood, it can continue to impair parenting.

Parents with troubled family-of-origin histories often have unrealistic notions, clinging to romantic ideas of being the perfect parent. Without an internal road map for what's normal, they don't realize how much adversity naturally exists, even in the happiest of families. They panic when their teens mouth off, pitch fits, and hate them when they don't get their way. Haunted by their past and too focused on being loved and cherished, such parents fear a bad relationship with their child and buckle, even if they "know" better in their rational minds. This description may sound extreme, but many of today's parents get overwhelmed by their children's hissy fits. When kids whine and protest, "That's not fair," parents commonly talk too much, engage too much, and defend too much, trying too hard to fix it when their kids are unhappy with them.

Pathways to Indulgence

Children are "indulged" when they have too many resources and not enough responsibility. In other words, the benefits they're receiving from parents are out of proportion with what they're doing to earn them. This can happen when parents set such a high priority on athletics, grades, and talent development that there is precious little time left for the difficult agenda of enforcing drudgery. These parents are pushovers when their adolescents whine that they have a paper to write and can't do the dishes.

"Spoiling" comes about for many reasons, not just because of boundary or family-of-origin problems. American culture and social circumstances impact many families.

Common causes of indulgence:

- Financial: Parents today have more disposable income to put toward children's wish lists.
- Demographic: Parents are having fewer children and having them later, which means less divvying up of resources.
- Slippery slope: Kids love stuff, we love our kids, we fall into the bad habit of giving them stuff because we love to see those faces shine.
- Guilt: We give them stuff instead of time.
- Overwhelmed by the intensity: Teens' increased sensitivity to the pleasure hormone (dopamine) means they can come after parents with a vengeance when they don't get what they want.
- The "busy" excuse: Our kids are too busy and so are we, and we never get around to making chores a priority.
- Overidentification: "I want them to have what I didn't from my childhood."
- Pure "oops": We get into the habit of giving them stuff and didn't realize where all those "gimmes" would end up.
- Path of least resistance: It's easier to do household chores yourself or hire them out than to make kids do them.
- Retail therapy: You're having a bad day and give yourself a boost by treating the kids and enjoying making them happy.
- Misguided self-esteem: We feel more successful when we provide our kids with more.
- Hitting a rough patch in life: Any tough time—divorce, illness, difficult circumstances—can lower a parent's resistance to kids' demands.
- Our material world: Almost everyone is tempted to "keep up with the Joneses."
- Exhaustion: Parents are on a treadmill, too tired to summon up the strength to hold the line.

Indulging children is only too easy. What's hard is sticking to our guns and making it a priority in our busy lives to teach children the skills they need to delay gratification, budget resources, and be responsible members of the family. Highly indulged kids are not happy kids. Children who get by on feeling good because they have things, without making strong efforts and developing competencies, typically have a false, inflated sense of importance, which is inversely related to genuine self-esteem.

Happy kids work toward achieving goals. Research shows that a strong sense of self develops when kids experience tough but surmountable challenges, buckle down, and learn to overcome them. Having supportive parents in the background helps the process. Teens may be grouchy and grumpy when we insist on chores. They may be disappointed when we deny them their desires. But parents who cave to their teen's demands are robbing them of the chance to develop habits of personal responsibility that can take them far in the world.

Harsh though it may sound, kids can't become spoiled unless parents have a lenient parenting style and/or make errors in judgment in giving them too much stuff. Something for nothing isn't a life rule that advances any kind of positive child development. Occasions when we are supergenerous should stand out as a pleasant exception.

A spoiled teen is years in the making. Given how distasteful chores can be to kids, parents will need to brace themselves for how difficult and time consuming it will be to inculcate them. If parents have lapsed and kids aren't pulling their weight, a family overhaul will take considerable effort. Like any repair job, it will require careful attention to a lot of areas as well as significant teamwork. Unless parents hang together, children may pick off the weaker parent, creating discord if the stronger parent turns on the one who capitulates.

No teen wants to be a spoiled brat, but they want what they want. During the teen years, they thank us for the wrong things—letting them get out of chores and giving them stuff. A decade down the line, older kids will likely express gratitude to parents who raised them to clean up their own messes and pull their own weight. Only years later will they appreciate the character strengths developed by being held responsible for tasks as mundane as mowing the lawn, washing the car, or earning their own money for a dazzling new goody.

CHAPTER 6

When You're Worried You're Losing Your Teen

What Am I, Chopped Liver?

A mom buys her 13-year-old daughter the next book in a series that she's reading, expecting the usual smile and appreciative hug.

Mom: I picked this up for you today. I'll bet you can't wait to read it. It's my turn next!
Daughter: I don't read that anymore.
Mom: But you were up until all hours of the night reading the last one.
Daughter: Those books are stupid. You like them, I don't.

What's going on? This is a classic teen declaration of independence. Mom is assuming that her daughter is the same person she was six months ago—or even last week—with the same preferences in clothes, food, activities, and music. Teens don't want to be clones of their parents. They wrestle with their identities relative to their parents in a process called "individuation." When teens join the new tribe of adolescence, they can bite off a parent's head whenever their mom or dad presumes to know their tastes. They're defending their precious and fledgling selves, as if to say, "You think you know me, but you don't at all."

A 12-year-old daughter is having a small slumber party, and a mom decides to make cookies for the girls. As they're baking, she ducks her head into her daughter's bedroom.

Mom: I've got some chocolate chip cookies in the oven for you girls. I'll bring them up while they're still warm with some cocoa.
Daughter: Don't bother.
Mom: Oh, it's no problem. I made them for you. They'll be yummy!
Daughter: We don't need cookies, Mom. We just need some privacy.

What's going on? Deep down, teens still love, respect, and value their parents, but at this stage of the game, they feel crowded by the mere presence of their parents. They need to assert and protect their new territory, which includes not only rooms and friends but their expanding psychological and social worlds. As they try on new selves, they don't want their parents around, and may be willing to sacrifice something they love, particularly around friends. Privacy is the way that teens put distance between their parents and themselves.

It's dinner time and a mom is serving up one of her 14-year-old son's favorites, her special lasagna.

Mom: I hope you're hungry. I made lasagna with chicken.

Son: You should taste Charlie's mom's lasagna. It's incredible.

Mom: I thought you liked the way I made it.

Son: Oh, she's the best cook in the world.

What's going on? Teens deliver big "ouches" like this, not to offend but to overturn the status quo. During adolescence, parents are "dethroned." Young children get angry with their parents when they don't get their way or are disappointed, but mom and dad are still pretty much heroes, and moments of adoration are more apparent. In order to "dethrone" their parents, teens go out of their way to elevate someone else, which serves to put parents down and make more room for the teens' budding selves.

Selfhood 2.0

Most parents have at least a nodding appreciation for "identity exploration" during adolescence. No matter how readily this term is tossed around to explain a boatload of changes in teens—new hair, clothes, music, language, room decoration, emotional distancing—we can still underestimate how taxing this process can be for everyone in the family. Moreover, we don't always appreciate what a profound and multidimensional concept "identity" is. Not one thing, identity consists of a bundle of internal and external dimensions, including feelings, ideas, values, preferences, ethnicity, personality, spirituality, gender, sexuality, appearance, work, and lifestyle. Sorting all this out and re-integrating it into a smoothly running, updated self is a mind-boggling process.

Exploration of identity is the big agenda item in adolescents' lives. Teens are the epitome of a work in process in identity building. With their identities under construction, they can be very self-conscious, defensive, and wobbly in their bearings during middle school and much of high school. The adolescent years usher in significant changes, not only for teens, but also for parents whose own identities are tweaked in the process.

Young children show their appreciation for parents more overtly, but with tweens and teens, a new attitude unfolds. We shift from "I'm the parent of the little cutie cuddling with me" to "I'm the parent of the sullen kid with a shaggy hair, saggy pants, and bad posture." Parents can grieve over no longer having a young son or daughter who imitates them, wants to be their "buddy," and is compliant most of the time.

Adding insult to injury, some teens peck away at parents, critiquing them for things as miniscule as the way they talk, laugh, dress, or even eat a sandwich. Pecking arises from a perfect storm, as circumstance and biology swirl together. Here's what's brewing:

- Because of their age and stage, teens are off center and uncertain in their own identities.
- Teens need to individuate (meaning establish their individuality or unique self) and be "not my parents."
- Teens' new brains give them analytic abilities to see all our flaws and shortcomings. They're up, we're down.
- Since they're still closest to us, we're the safest targets on which they can inflict their bad moods. Although also true of young children, teens go out of their way to create friction with parents, which allows them to keep a distance and see us in a negative light.
- As part of child rearing, we've been after our teens for years to "Put on a good shirt . . . Leave your muddy shoes outside . . . Go to bed, it's a school night . . . Don't slouch . . . Chew with your mouth closed." Although all for good reasons, it's oppressive enough to motivate them to retaliate with little digs.

Here's an example of where this can lead: A mom explains to her family that dinner will be late, saying, "I spent all afternoon with Grandma at the doctor's office." The teen son butts in to correct Mom, "Why are you always exaggerating? It was only three hours." The mom hasn't done anything to deserve this nasty remark, but here is a son who is wobbly himself, being in the middle of the separation process, yet is eagle-eyed about his mom's imperfections, in a bad mood because he is hungry, and feels regularly needled by mom. Now he can use his clever new brain not only to get back at Mom for her history of requests and demands, but to throw her off kilter, too.

Parents can be taken aback by teen aggression and negativity. If they fail to grasp the big picture and desirability of the Selfhood 2.0 process, they could easily work up a negative attitude of their own to match that of their teen. No wonder there can be so much negativity all around in families during the adolescent years.

As part of their arduous journey of identity, teens seek privacy. Although parents can feel wounded and disoriented by this demand, a degree of distancing assures teens that the self they are forging is truly theirs and, importantly, they avoid our judgments. Keeping parents at arm's length lets teens question our values and explore fragile new ideas (which they may not act on) through conversations with friends or in their journals.

Even from week to week, teens may slip into something new and then do an about-face. A teen girl might, for example, try out using foul language with peers and develop a crush and flirt with a teen with a bad reputation. In her own time, she might determine that this foray over to the dark side doesn't feel right. The last thing she needs is her parents panicking and over-reacting to something she's testing out, particularly since she sees it as harmless and her business, not theirs.

Identity development occurs in the nooks and crannies of a self, as teens ponder small decisions that will accumulate and add up to "This is who I am": "Should I go to the school dance or sacrifice this fun thing to go to my soccer play-offs?" "Should I do trail conservation this summer like my parents want or work on my DJ spinning?" "Should I stand up to that bossy, popular kid, even if it makes me unpopular?" "Should I raise my hand and risk being seen as a nerd in class when I know the answers but others don't?" "Is it phony of me to be nice to kids I don't really want to be friends with?"

Adults make parallel judgment calls day in and day out, but we choose one option over the other by using our established blueprints. Not mature enough to be decisive, teens agonize as if the world depended on it. With so much at stake during the creation of Selfhood 2.0, small wonder that teens spend hours preoccupied with their own worlds.

The Self-Centeredness of Young Teens

Teen's action	Parent's assumption	In teen's mind
13-year-old leaves used, wet towels in her bedroom and just gets another clean one next time, creating more laundry.	*She is lazy, selfish, and inconsiderate, not remembering what she's been told a million times.*	*I'm just busy. I resent what a big deal my parent is making about this when it's just a towel, and she's making me feel like a bad person.*
12-year-old has a meltdown and refuses to go to school because of a very large, unattractive zit on his nose.	*This is sheer vanity. A little cover-up and hardly anyone will notice. He needs to cope better than this and not be so sensitive to what others think.*	*If I go to school, everyone will notice my acne and tease me. All I'll be able to think about is this huge zit, and they'll all be thinking the same thing, too.*

Teen's action	Parent's assumption	In teen's mind
12-year-old insists on being dropped off two blocks away from a movie, shouting urgently, "Stop here, stop here!"	*How rude not to thank me and how silly for her to pretend she got here any other way since I drive her everywhere.*	*It makes me look like a baby to be driven around. I feel like a loser being seen with my parents.*
13-year-old ignores homework to spend his time practicing with his band so he can make a recording and become a rock star.	*Talk about delusions of grandeur! He's not thinking logically about what his chances are of making it in the competitive music industry.*	*Why can't my parents just believe in me? I'm good. I don't need school. When I make my first recording, someone will notice and sign me on. My parents will be sorry.*

In each situation, the teen might say, "My parents just don't get it!" but the parent would retort, "Well, neither do you!" Both are a little bit right, but they might as well be speaking different languages. Developmental psychologists, however, have a word to describe the teen's behavior: "egocentrism," meaning "the center of my psychological world is me."

Although parents may experience egocentrism as selfishness, it's part of a teen's developmental stage. Between brain maturation and the intricacies of figuring out a self, there will be kinks in the system. We shouldn't expect a reconfigured self to be up and running with new and old values synchronized overnight. Some years hence, teens can become independent, high functioning, and ready to launch into the world, but this complex process will necessarily have hiccups.

Self-absorbed, preoccupied, and wound up in themselves, young adolescents of about ages 12 to 14 live in little "all about me" bubbles, a condition that may not be resolved until around age 16. At any point in time, they may have a separate reality playing in their heads, as they muse over their science test, their complexion, their friendships, their play list, and the teacher who hates them. Selfies posted on a favorite social media site abet the manufacturing and curating of an identity a teen wants but doesn't necessarily have.

With their higher-level brain functions still under construction, teens' immature brains can't always process the bigger picture of their predicament.

When parents confront teens on their thoughtlessness, selfishness, or irrationality, parents may hit a wall of protest, fury, or rigid resistance. And if parents' emotional brains are activated at the same time as the teens', sparks can really fly. During such conflicts, we can remind ourselves of one of the cardinal rules of "getting to calm": Don't talk when you're under the influence of intense emotion.

As the above situations bear out, egocentrism drives parents to distraction, mainly because of the following characteristics.

Teens at this stage aren't always aware of how their behavior is going to impact others. Many teen screw-ups—like leaving wet towels around—can appear defiant. Parents often assign bad motives to actions that are better described as forms of inattentiveness rather than flagrant rule breaking. Preoccupied with their new bodies, thoughts, future fantasies, and daily experiences, they have a dozen items that are higher priorities than being a good citizen according to Mom and Dad.

They think that everyone is looking at them all the time and judging them as harshly as they do themselves. The boy with the blemish suffers from what is sometimes called an "imaginary audience." Incredibly self-conscious, teens at this phase feel as if they are on a stage with everyone watching. They have trouble separating their own thoughts from those of others. Their reality is everyone's reality. Likewise, the girl who is mortified to be seen with her parent feels the glare of the spotlight. Because she feels like a kindergartener being driven around by her parents, everyone else must be laughing about it behind her back.

They spend an inordinate amount of time in their heads spinning possibilities, including fantastic dreams and worst-case nightmares. Young children have the imagination to pretend they're a ballerina, Superman, or a black belt in karate, but with teens it's not "pretend," it's "if/then, if/then." Capable of hypothetical thinking, they can plan and analyze the steps along the way. But because they're in a bubble, they're not always tethered to reality. Traveling into unexplored mental territory with their new brains, they plot future schemes, as with the boy who is convinced he is headed to L.A. to be the next big rock star. Mental tripping can consume hours.

Teens will grow out of egocentrism, especially if parents play their cards right by avoiding power struggles, which make teens keep up their resistance to parents' controlling ways. By the time teens reach 15 or 16, they can usually tune into others' ideas—not just their own—and figure out how they're coming across. Less myopic, they can reflect, put things in perspective, and adjust their behavior.

In the meantime, however, parents suffer at the hands of their teen's egocentric behavior. We probably don't want to wait around until they grow out of it. Plus, part of our role is to nudge them into being decent, considerate, thoughtful members of society, as overbearing as that can sometimes seem to them.

What to do, then, about a young teen's inconsiderate acts? The good news is that we don't need to become morally indignant. Not necessarily a sign of "bad character," these behaviors are in line with normal adolescence. The bad news is that these behaviors can be the bane of our existence: "He's upstairs staring in the mirror, changing his clothes, while I put his books in his backpack so he won't miss the bus!" or "She borrowed my best sweater, claiming she would value it with her life, but at the end of the day, I found it crumpled in a corner of her room!"

The key is not to get tangled up emotionally with teens, carrying on and brow-beating them. It's as if parents want the teen to cry uncle, admit she has been self-centered, rude, selfish, and bad. This is asking way too much of a wobbly, emotionally fragile kid.

We should make our point precisely: "Stop changing your clothes and get your backpack ready to go now, please." Period. "I'm angry that my good sweater is on the floor in your room. I expect you to pay to have it dry-cleaned." Period. Keep it simple and to the point. And, of course, it requires a calm mind to remember the advantages of brevity.

In nonjudgmental terms, we can tell them how their behavior has impacted us. "I'm fuming. You forgot to put the roast in the oven, so we're going to be late for the meeting. Think about it." Limit responses to two or three sentences maximum, steering clear of words like "thoughtless" and "selfish." The question for parents should be "What is the chance that saying more will help or hurt the point I need to make?" Piling on leads to overkill, not greater insights and changed behavior in the teen.

Imposing a natural consequence that speaks for itself ("pay to clean the sweater") or responding succinctly keeps the heat on the teenager. When we blast away at our kids, we steal our own thunder and undermine our goal of helping them see the consequences of their behavior. What our kids register is how mean and out of control we are.

Peer relationships are a potent force in moving teens away from their self-focus. All day long, in countless interactions, teens are telling it like it is: "You jerk. You forgot to call me back." "How selfish can you get?" "Stop hogging the ball." "You were really showing off." "You're too sensitive." "You stare at yourself in the mirror a lot." Or the number-one piece of feedback among girls, "All you do is talk about yourself."

Challenges like these help adolescents see how they're experienced by others. Though it can get vicious, some little jabs from peers are worth their weight in gold. Peers can be parents' allies in the "anti-egocentrism" cause, but we hardly ever credit them. As we compete with peers for time and influence, we sometimes forget that we're not the only member of the team helping our teens move beyond "me, me, me."

Lie Low and Wear Beige

Back in the simpler years of childrearing, our grade-schoolers welcomed us into their classrooms and hugged us in the presence of peers. But during early adolescence, every word out of a parent's mouth can be a source of embarrassment to their child. Make a silly gesture, crack a joke or—heaven forbid—do something remotely flamboyant in front of friends, and they cringe, sulk, or call us "lame." What a slap in the face it is when parents can't be themselves anymore!

Here's an example: Driving a carpool with his 12-year-old daughter, a dad turns the radio to a country music station and begins singing along. The daughter abruptly switches the station and asks him to stop. Because he thinks he's being funny, he returns to the country station and resumes crooning, adding more flair to his solo. Although the friends are laughing, the daughter is in a huff. "Where's your sense of humor?' he laughs, trying to keep things light. Angry and humiliated, the daughter clams up and averts her steely gaze out the car window. Dad is stupefied.

Here's advice for this dad: Lie low and wear beige. Parents of middle-school students, particularly parents with strong personalities, may need to tone it way down for a few years. Touchy and highly self-conscious, young teens like this daughter are worried they're not cool enough around friends. In the best of times she finds her dad mildly irritating, but as he upstages her around friends, his imperfections are magnified in her mind, and now he's ruining her chances of being popular.

Dad is just "doing his thing," but she's thinking, "These are my friends. This should be about 'my thing.'" Even if friends think we're hilarious, reality doesn't matter. What matters is our teen's experience that we're obnoxious and stealing the show. Remember, as parents we're the big oak tree, shading their growth. Before we even open our mouths, we're oppressive, but add any overt personality and we're asking to be chopped down. For some parents, it's worth it to "just be myself," but they should at least be aware of the risk. Down the line, when this daughter is less merged with her parent and more secure in her separate self, she'll be able to shrug off Dad's singing, saying, "That's my dad. He's silly sometimes."

Like this dad, parents worry that their teens have lost their sense of humor. Around friends, teens are hyper-concerned about how they're being perceived. In an agitated state, they're carrying lots of emotion. The smart move for parents is to stay neutral, because a teen's big magnifying lens will detect and exaggerate our quirks. If parents stick their necks out and display a colorful personality, teens can become openly hostile, expressing their burgeoning Selfhood 2.0 by being rude.

"Chest beating" in front of friends is a public display of a teen's new independence. Starting with the middle-school years and into high school, there will be a huge reduction in the number of warm, easygoing interactions we have with our children, particularly around peers. At times, they might be back for a cuddle, but it's still not easy when our children have more complicated feelings toward us.

Family Story: A Dad Struggles With His Son's Choices

Until recently, adolescence in the Bauer household had been smooth sailing—no radical piercings, no beer bottles in the back of the closet, no major challenges to family expectations. The oldest son in the family, 16-year-old Gregory, was even-tempered, mature for his age, a good student, and the apple of his father's eye as a basketball player, Dad's favorite sport.

The only little ripple occurred when Gregory started going out with a flamboyant girlfriend, whom Irvin, Gregory's father, gruffly declared was "too artsy." Sharon, Gregory's mom, tried to make the point that it was Gregory's girlfriend, not his father's, but Dad carped nonstop until the girlfriend was history.

Though Irvin was a domineering dad giving the family their marching orders, Gregory was smart enough to stay under the radar screen and keep his ideas to himself. Mom likewise felt that it was easier to go with the flow, agree with Dad, and maintain harmony in the home.

For a dad who thinks he's always right, Irvin was dealt a huge blow when Gregory told him that he'd gotten the lead in the school play and was giving up basketball. Irvin vehemently opposed this decision. Realizing theater was where her son's heart was, Sharon, for the first time, questioned Irvin's judgment.

Discussions between dad and son on this issue became hotter and hotter. One evening, deciding he'd heard enough, Gregory headed out the door. Irvin stepped in front of him saying, "I'm talking to you, son! You stay right here!" When Gregory kept going, his dad tried to hold him by the shoulder, and the situation nearly came to blows. The fight distressed everyone. No one could believe that this could happen in their family. Shaken up, they decided to visit a psychologist for a consultation.

What follows is an excerpt from the Bauer family's initial session with author Laura Kastner:

Dad (Irvin): I'm just saying that sometimes parents can have greater wisdom about how a decision might play out down the line than a teenager.

Gregory: Dad, you think you know what's best for me, but you don't. I'm a mediocre basketball player on a mediocre team. I can't see how this makes such a difference in my college "options," as you call them.

Dad: Now, Gregory, you never know how much you can mature into the game, especially with extra training. And you haven't even hit your full growth spurt. Basketball could be just the tip to help you get into a top school if you really work at it. Let's face it—theater is fun, but not on par with sports in the college admissions game.

(Gregory rolls his eyes, giving the impression that they've covered this ground many times.)

Mom (Sharon, addressing Kastner): This is the disagreement that led to the showdown last week.

Kastner: Mr. Bauer, I'm assuming that for you to end up in such a heated altercation over this issue, you have very strong concerns about Gregory dropping basketball in order to participate in this play.

Dad: Yes, I think it is a mistake. And I was upset that he kept his audition for the play a secret. That was very underhanded of him after all the support I've given him and his team over the years.

Gregory: I didn't tell you because I knew you would flip out! And you did!

Kastner: Mr. Bauer, what are your deepest fears about Gregory pursuing theater instead of basketball?

Dad: My concern is that Gregory is making a mistake. With some effort, Gregory could be a strong basketball player. He just needs to apply himself. Isn't this what parents are supposed to do? Guide their children on tough decisions?

Gregory: Guide? You mean dictate!

Mom: I guess that's the problem. We need to figure out whose decision this is — ours or Gregory's.

Dad: Yes. And the other problem is how you and Gregory have been talking about this behind my back. (He looks at Kastner.) Aren't parents supposed to stand together? I was excluded from the play audition, and it hit me like a ton of bricks!

Mom: Really, Irvin, you've known how much Gregory has loved theater for years! It's just that until now, his participation never directly competed with basketball. The crux of this is that you've loved his school basketball as much as he has — actually, more!

Kastner: Mrs. Bauer, how would you describe the way you and your husband have operated around the hot topics of sports, theater, and Gregory's right to make decisions in these arenas?

Mom: Well, you see, my husband is used to being in a leadership position — at work, in Gregory's sports, and as head of the parent athletic support committee at school. Gregory's preference for theater over basketball has come as a rude awakening for Irvin. However, I think if he had been listening to Gregory, he would have known. Irvin is taking this hard. He's a "command and control" kind of guy. He's not used to defiance.

Gregory: Oh, great, all I did was audition for a play. And now I'm being defiant.

Mom: I'm sorry, Gregory. I didn't mean it that way. What I meant was that I usually go along with your dad on things, and yet on this one, I just can't. (She looks to Kastner.) I must admit it — I think Gregory should make the choice, but Irvin believes that I'm wrong and that leaving our son to his own choice is cheating him out of a parent's wisdom.

Kastner: Gregory, can you tell me when you respect his "command and control" style?

Gregory: His "take charge" approach can be great for some stuff—like the way he gets sponsors for the athletic equipment at school—but when you disagree, forget about it. That's why I auditioned without telling him. I was just postponing the blow-up. I didn't know I'd get the lead. He's the one who loves basketball, not me.

Forks in the Road: Who Gets to Choose the Way?

Irvin's decisive, action-oriented style helped him grow his own successful small business and, likewise, served the community well when it came to goals like raising money for the school's athletic program. A dedicated dad, he put enormous energy into the family, kept the household train running on time, and set the bar high for family achievement. Everything was proceeding according to plan until his authoritarian style smacked headlong into his son's identity development.

Every personal strength can have an underbelly. Irvin ruled the roost capably, but he hadn't learned how to accommodate family members' opposing ideas. Used to having his way, he didn't know how to negotiate differences and solve problems. Although his argument about basketball and college admissions came across as reasonable enough, in this emotionally arousing crisis, he was practically shoving basketball down his son's throat.

Cheerful and easygoing, Sharon had held things together by not challenging Irvin. Her sweet, genial nature was a strength, but it carried a downside. Like many women, Sharon was raised to be nice and steer clear of conflict. Over the years, she avoided confronting Irvin on issue after issue, giving way to his preferences for vacation choices, whom to socialize with, where to shop, how to spend money, and so on. In her mind, this was a virtue, because it kept the home warm and pleasant, but by always accommodating Irvin, she let him stay a bulldog.

Irvin hadn't developed any of the qualities that make intimate relationships work, such as listening to and acknowledging others' positions, being empathetic, and collaborating. Not having blazed the way, Sharon left it to her son to be the one to take on the big guy.

As the Bauer family's dilemma illustrates, teen identity development can upset the applecart, overturning everyone's role and interaction in the family dynamic.

From their family story, here are some take-away points:

When families meet at a developmental crossroads, watch out for collisions. Teen identity decisions hit different parents differently. Whether it's a daughter getting a navel piercing or son mouthing a radical opinion at

the dinner table, how we experience our children's identity exploration is a reflecting pool for our own values, temperaments, and life experience. Trouble always brews when parents see a teen's identity choice as "going against them."

After many years of pleasing Dad and playing basketball, Gregory is lighting out for new identity territory. Mom, meanwhile, has life issues of her own to consider. With Gregory nearing the end of high school, Sharon has reached her own developmental transition of wanting to "individuate" from her husband's autocratic rule at the same time as her teen. Many wives won't break out of the role of pleaser with their domineering husbands for themselves, but they can become mother-bear crusaders for their children.

Irvin was more than content with business as usual, but others' actions drove him to a developmental crossroads with numerous losses to face. Gone are his wife's and son's compliance that had made his life easier. He must deal with the ego-bruising reality of Gregory's preference for theater. He'll no longer have the satisfaction of championing his beloved basketball, and on top of it all, he'll soon be confronting the loss of parenting his son day to day when Gregory heads to college.

Irvin is up against hard lessons about sharing power. But if he opens himself up, he stands to gain far more than the loss of his "command and control" seat. He can gain more intimacy and trust with his loved ones.

Teens' identity decisions can hit parents at a gut level.
When Irvin moved to restrain Gregory physically, his emotional brain registered that his son was making a catastrophic decision. Circuits blew: Failure! Mistake! Blowing his chances at a good life! Defiance! Disrespect! Humiliation among my friends and colleagues!

Irvin had never been in the position where he needed to take the proverbial deep breath to calm himself and see the folly of his overreaction, because Gregory had been compliant in every way. Whether it's music, clothing, or choice of room décor, many teen tastes and preferences make parents uncomfortable, sometimes extremely so. With the irrationality of road rage, parents can take on every choice they don't agree with as over the top.

Wise parents leave harmless choices alone and carefully select the ones they decide to trump. Let's say, for example, that after some deliberation, a parent realizes she can't go along her teen's highly sexualized clothes. If this is the case, she can approach her teen in a humble way, even with an apology, saying, "I'm sorry that I'm overriding your choices. I don't think it's appropriate for you to be wearing that shirt. It's too revealing, it sexualizes your presentation to the world, and I'm not comfortable with it even though you are." Discussions on sensitive issues like this (and most identity decisions are sensitive) might not go well, but a calm, thoughtful assessment stands a better chance of reaching the teen than a knee-jerk reaction.

Despite all the things we desperately want for our teens, their lives aren't supposed to be all about us. What if our kids stayed little clones of us instead of forging their own ways? What if Gregory went along with his dad and stayed on the basketball team, never giving theater a shot? Irvin wouldn't experience it as a loss, but Gregory would.

Depriving a teen of the Selfhood 2.0 process means less self-exploration of skills, less awareness of future paths of fulfillment, less happiness, and less building of a unique identity. Our children's selfhood isn't supposed to be about us. Often our "wise" opinions are nothing more than our projections of what we want to be true, good, and desirable for our teens. Since we are not our children, and we don't have crystal balls for seeing exactly whom they're supposed to become, we all need to practice humility in matters of their identity choices, interests, beliefs, and desires. Matters of safety, risk taking, and other behavioral areas are different, and that's where we want to weigh in.

Many parents have to work hard to make peace with the person their child turns out to be, especially when it's at odds with their own identities and dreams for their child.

Identity Development: There's a Method to the Madness
Too easily, parents get pulled into battles over behaviors that are harmless, superficial, or just a testing of the waters, instead of saving nonnegotiable decisions for crucial matters.

Studies have looked at adolescents' shifting values around important areas of sexuality, religion, political views, and careers. Starting in middle school, teens sift through the leanings of their parents and peers as well as the ideas around them, ultimately arriving at their own set of values in their twenties. Generally speaking, teens go out a distance from their parents as they form their identities, then circle back in the direction of the values they were brought up with.

While teens may adopt the styles and tastes of their peers, they're unlikely to relinquish learned ethical principles related to right versus wrong (lying, cheating, or stealing, for example). Research on educational and career choices shows that parents' influence outweighs that of peers. Although peers have a bearing on teens' experimentation with risky behaviors, such as sex and substance use, parents can mediate this influence, as can social/cultural groups (schools, neighborhoods, and religious institutions, for example).

In general, identity development during the teen years involves examining new ideas, committing to some and throwing out others along the way, and ultimately weaving together a storyline of "who I am" over time.

The progression looks something like this:

1. *I'm just like you.*
Note to parents: Enjoy this first decade of life, because this "clone" stage is not supposed to last.

2. *I'm anything but you—I think.*
Note to parents: Don't get too reactive during this experimental stage, because it could change by next week.

3. *I am committed to new beliefs and want you to respect them.*
Note to parents: Watch out for bashing their ideologies, because in essence, you'll be bashing them.

4. *I'm mostly me, but there is a lot of you in me, too.*
Note to parents: Don't be surprised at the degree to which your kids end up having values similar to yours. By their early twenties, most will have integrated a set of views reflecting their personal journeys, their parents' beliefs, and the customs of their generation of peers.

Culture plays an important role in how the stages play out, especially for people of color and for families that are strongly identified with a specific cultural background. Despite the diversity of the U.S. population, teens want to belong to their teen tribe, and media has a way of brainwashing kids into being what is "cool." This exposure can threaten parents' hopes of instilling respect for family heritage. There's no recipe for ensuring that a teen adopts his parents' cultural identity, given the intrinsic desire of teenagers to be independent thinkers. We help our kids establish positive cultural and racial identities through stories, rituals, and relationships with people we think will inspire them with appreciation for their culture.

Almost all parents get perturbed when their teens express views that run counter to their own ideologies. Let's say, for example, that a son expresses the opinion that not only should marijuana be legalized at the federal level, but that the legal age should be 14. His parents couldn't disagree more. How should they handle this?

If a parent and a teen are having an interesting and positive interchange, in which everyone is articulating views, listening, and staying respectful, it's a good thing. But if the discussion gets heated and degenerates, there's no purpose in keeping it up. Sometimes, teens become provocative and saucy to get a parent's goat. Parents can wig out and try to convince their teens they're wrong, as if to say, "I know the world. I know you. I know what's best. Let me persuade you to feel differently."

Studies validate an approach in which parents stay calm and unthreatened. Research shows that parents who listen, acknowledge, share their own views—but don't criticize or try to persuade their teen to abandon their views—will have more competent, well-adjusted teens.[1] Accepting and respecting teens' personal thoughts and feelings are the key contributions to healthy identity development.

Within certain parameters, individuation from parents is not only natural but desirable. Teens who stay at the "I'm like you" stage remain stunted versions of themselves. As farfetched as it may seem, parents should be able to look at their teens' shaggy hair or ankle tattoo and think, "I want this, because I know it's better for them to go through an exploration of self, values, and choices than to remain closed off." Research shows that teens who have struggled, differentiated from their parents, and become committed to their own positive selves are more ethical, empathetic, and well adjusted than kids who are low in identity achievement.[2] Moreover, they're willing to assume more personal responsibility for themselves and their world. For everything we dislike about the Selfhood 2.0 process, the outcome can knock our socks off.

When teens trade in the clothes, music, language, and ways of their youth to be more in tune with their peers, parents can feel bewildered and alarmed, because many of these changes stand for a loss of childhood. Fragile, self-conscious, and self-absorbed as they form their new selves, teens can put their parents through the wringer with their shifting identities. Be it our religion, political party, or educational goals, when our teens question values we consider sacred ground, we can become more distressed than at any other time of our lives.

Like learning to walk and talk, identity building is a developmental process. But unlike walking and talking, which are full of joy and fun despite a stumble or two, identity seeking can be messy and unpleasant, and the necessary stumbles can be more harmful and scary. Parents of older children can be a source of reassurance. The great majority will report that the outcome of the selfhood growth process—stormy though it may be—is more wondrous and satisfying than ever imagined.

CHAPTER 7

When They're Screaming at You — or Not Talking at All

Teens are prickly for various reasons, but a good parent-child relationship reduces the odds against any number of big-ticket problems such as mental-health issues, extreme risk taking, and school failure. Having a good relationship means keeping lines of communication open, listening well, staying positive, using authority wisely, and picking your battles. Being aware of what we "should" do to keep a positive connection is one thing, but the reality of pulling it off is another. Let's take the mother-daughter duo first.

Mothers and daughters struggle in ways that differ from mother-son conflicts or father-son conflicts, which have their own masculine mystery. Mothers and daughters fight more than any other parent-child pair, quarreling twice as much as mothers and sons. One study documented the staying power of mother-daughter sparring: Compared to mother-son arguments, which tend to last about six minutes, mothers and daughters stay engaged for about 15 minutes.[1]

Even calm, cool, and collected moms will occasionally lose it and get into skirmishes with their frenzied daughters. Despite how irrational they may seem, conflicts between mothers and daughters aren't struggles over nonsense. Very often, low-boil squabbling serves an important function. Going after Mom is a girl's bid to individuate and gain recognition as a different, competent, and unique person. Through bickering, girls can affirm that they are separate selves, and the more exaggerated the conflict, the greater the assurance that "I'm not anything like my mom."[2]

Fighting is not necessarily a measure of a bad relationship between a mom and daughter. Moms can be very hurt by what comes across as a form of rejection, but when surveyed later, many girls who quarreled regularly with their moms say they have a close, supportive, and valued relationship. In other words, daughters are spoiling for a fight in order to separate, but they still want the connection.

Family Story: A Savvy Mom Avoids a Mother-Daughter Tornado

Arguments between mothers and teenage daughters may be as regular as rain, but when the twosome is a high-strung, reactive mother and a high-strung, pubescent daughter, it can look so crazy that dads are mystified by the emotional downpour. Because mothers, more so than fathers, tend to listen to their daughters' problems and complaints, they're more easily swept into the turmoil. Dads may be sympathetic, but they usually have a lower tolerance for emotionality.

Why are some moms and daughters able to contain their quarrels, while others routinely get drawn into big fights that spin out of control? Various factors come into play to determine the intensity of the quarreling. Mother-daughter duos with the very lowest risk for big tussles have this set of characteristics:

- Both mother and daughter have calm temperaments.
- There are no social stressors, such as boyfriend blues, financial problems, marital strains, or parent illness.
- Both mother and daughter have hormones in balance and are in good health.
- Good social support is available.
- Boundaries are firm.
- Mom has no significant family-of-origin issues (early loss of a parent, a wayward sibling, for example) to trigger high emotions.

Problems with any of these variables can spark big fights. Take, for instance, a mom who had a difficult, conflict-filled, highly reactive relationship with her own mom (her "family of origin"). Put her together with a daughter who is PMS-ing at the same time as the mom, and it's a powder keg waiting to blow.

In the following tussle between 16-year-old Sheri and her mother, Louise, the salient factor is the daughter's tightly wound temperament. The upside of her temperament is that she sets rigorous standards for herself, excelling in school and sports, and presenting an impressive face to the world. At home, however, she is a highly emotional teen, easily agitated and easily upset. Over the years, Louise has learned how readily things can escalate with her daughter unless she keeps her composure.

Louise has just arrived home. In hand is a sweater from the dry cleaner's that she and Sheri previously discussed as a good choice for school pictures. As undesirable and difficult as this mother-daughter exchange is, it shows a mom doing her best in a tough situation.

What Sheri and her mom say:	**What each thinks:**
Mom (Louise): Here's the blue sweater you wanted for picture day tomorrow.	*Last year was such a scene when she got her pictures back. I really didn't have time to go to the clean-*

What Sheri and her mom say:

What each thinks:

ers, *but I was glad to do it because she is so self-conscious about her looks and body.*

Sheri: I'm not wearing that! I said "maybe." I don't know what I'm going to wear! I don't have anything good.

I'll feel like a stuffed pig in that sweater! I don't know what to wear. I'm so frustrated. I want my pictures to look really good this year.

Mom: What do you mean? We talked about how nice you look in it. It'll look great!

Oh, no . . . she is backing out on what I thought was settled. It's aggravating when she acts like she owns nothing "good" when she has a closet full of cute clothes.

Sheri (pitch rising): I don't want to wear it. Why are you shoving it at me like that? I never said I'd wear it! None of my clothes look right.

I'm going to look bad no matter what! I hate everything I own. Allison has everything she wants. Her pictures always turn out great. She's thin and beautiful. I hate the way I look. I hate my haircut. If I smile with my mouth closed, my lips pooch over my braces. If I smile big, my braces take over the whole picture.

Mom: I'm not shoving it at you, honey. It's just that I really think it will look lovely on you. Last year you were so upset about the plaid shirt clashing with your braces— that's why we talked about it last week.

I can see that Sheri is about to lose it here. No matter how much I reassure her, her emotions are making her feel like this is a monumental disaster. I probably need to just extract myself the best I can so she can settle down.

Sheri (whining): M-oooom! Take me to Allison's. Pl-ease. I talked to

Why won't she help me out here? I'm desperate. I don't know what

What Sheri and her mom say:

What each thinks:

her today at school, and she said she has a great idea for something I could borrow.

to wear. I hate that stupid sweater. Does she understand how important this is?

Mom: I'm sorry, Sheri. I am not going to drive you over to Allison's tonight. She's not at all your size, and the fit won't be right. But I don't expect you to accept my reasoning. I need to just have faith that you can figure out an alternative.

I need to be ready for one of Sheri's tizzies and know that I can't help solve her problem this minute. Just standing here invites a tirade because I'm seen as the problem now.

Sheri (starting to sound panicky): Another ugly picture! You just want me to wear the sweater because you don't want to take me to Allison's! You don't even care.

I can't stand how she won't listen. She thinks this is some stupid, petty thing. What do I have to do to show her how awful I feel? I just hate her.

Mom: Honey, I'm so sorry that you are unhappy with your options. I can see how important this is to you. School pictures are really, really important to teenagers. I wish there was an easy solution here, but mainly I think we need to cool off so that you can make a new plan. I'll come back in a while. I'm sorry I can't seem to help you.

I can't expect her to be anything but angry about my unwillingness to go to Allison's. I know that the best thing I can do at this point is to discontinue talking so that I don't make it worse.

Sheri (voice high pitched, tears welling up): There is an easy solution, Mom. Just take me to Allison's! Where are you going? Mom, don't walk away. Don't be that way!

She's not listening. I can't believe she is walking out on me. I feel like I'm going to explode. I'll call Allison and tell her what a bitch my mom is.

Although the situation went sideways in a nanosecond, this mom contained the upset as well as any parent with a cranked-up teen could. Even as Louise arrives home, Sheri is worked up about her pictures, ready to pounce on the first word out of Mom's mouth.

Louise can't help stating the obvious: Sheri isn't Allison's size. But she steers clear of sensitive comparisons about her daughter being "bigger" and avoids making volatile statements that would ratchet up the exchange like "How dare you speak to me like this!" or "Is this the thanks I get for going out of my way to get your sweater?"

The golden moment occurs when Louise realizes that Sheri is spinning out of control and there's little she can do to fix her daughter's upset. Louise has to nip it in the bud before it becomes a tirade, not by trying to solve or soothe, but by simply putting a stop to the conversation, as gracefully and gently as possible. By just standing there, she becomes a lightning rod for her daughter's anger; no matter what Louise says, she is going to be implicated in the problem.

Why was Louise able to remove herself deftly? Simply put: a healthy boundary. Louise can't put a stopper on her daughter's flooding emotions, but she can contain her own and avoid "co-flooding." Because her boundaries are firm instead of a sieve, Louise keeps Sheri's upset at bay and doesn't let it affect her judgment. A crucial skill of parenting an adolescent successfully is keeping your head when you're under attack. Louise accepts that Sheri may temporarily hate her, distort the situation completely, and set her up unfairly to be the "bad guy," but she realizes that all she can do is put a lid on the fire and exit before an even worse meltdown occurs.

Louise isn't being rigid about not taking Sheri to her friend's house. This isn't an option, since Allison's sweaters will be smaller sizes. It would be a futile effort to forestall an even more tempestuous situation an hour later when they're both more fatigued and the sweaters don't fit. Some situations don't have good options. The best you can do is cut your losses and keep your own part of the exchange clean.

Under the grip of her emotions, Sheri is physiologically aroused, and her heart is racing. If Louise had let the argument spiral, Sheri's heart rate would have continued to elevate, from, for example, 100 beats a minute or so to 130, and it could have become one of those huge rows where a daughter chases her mom down the hall, screaming at her through the locked bathroom door. Moms who react by keeping the fight alive and co-flooding with daughters build up a bad history of hurtful arguing. Once a mother and daughter establish a pattern of engaging together with high emotions, counseling may be the best option for changing habits and repairing the relationship.

Sheri and Louise's fight won't go there. True, they are both left with raw feelings, and Sheri feels like she hates her mom, but by curtailing the fight, Louise is also reining in the ill will. Louise and Sheri still have a good relationship. They'll be able to get back together later, and once Sheri calms down, she might even apologize.

Louise realizes that her daughter came out of the womb tightly wound. Especially during early adolescence, teen spinouts are sometimes hormonal and related to puberty, but Sheri's volatility also arises from her live-wire temperament. Once Sheri is older and has greater self-awareness, she'll be more capable of holding a mirror up to her behavior, critiquing herself, and restraining the emotions bubbling inside of her. For now though, mom has be the one to show her the way.

Dealing With Emotional Dumping

Fretful, overwrought teens don't want to be alone in their misery and will do everything in their power to pull their parents into their tempests, making parents miserable along with them. Parents rack their brains for a solution to make everything better, but it's important to be realistic. We can't keep our teens from having the misplaced motive of trying to engage us in their upsets. Empathy and support are critical to parenting, but there needs to be a balance: We don't want to let our teens use us as their emotional waste bin and, conversely, we don't want to leave them high and dry in their distress.

To achieve this delicate balance, there's a step-by-step process to follow whenever teens are cranked up for a fight and dumping for the sake of dumping. For high-strung teens, this can happen at any time, about anything, because the dynamic pertains more to the teen's frustration and anxiety than to any specific issue. Remember: Even if teens instigate an argument, grownups are responsible for bringing it to a halt.

With frantic teens, the tricky part is exiting while still staying positive. Using the CALM technique (Cool down; Assess options; Listen with empathy; Make a plan) and maintaining healthy boundaries can keep us thinking, instead of reacting and engaging in an escalating brouhaha. The process is teen-centric, meaning that we keep our own feelings out of the fray. The focus is on three goals:

- Keep emotions in check.
- Minimize damage to the relationship.
- Extricate ourselves from the eye of the storm.

Under most circumstances, we work to keep our teens sharing their ideas and feelings with us. Shutting them down just because we're weary of a little attitude is an ill-advised, aggressive ploy. But when a teen is emotionally "dys-regulated," experiencing flooding and extreme emotions, being rational isn't possible.

Here are the steps for removing yourself from the presence of a riled-up teen:

1. Listen, empathize, and confirm their feelings. A genuine and sincere tone is critical. If we're hovering or pandering ("I hear your feelings"), it can set the teen off. Instead, try a heartfelt comment like, "Wow, this sounds like a real struggle."

2. Admit you can't solve their problem. When someone is very upset, we're all tempted to try to solve the problem with our good advice. Unfortunately, this can come across as minimizing or patronizing, and can escalate the conflict. Instead, try something that pulls you away from their complaining cycle such as, "I'd love nothing more than to come up with a brilliant solution that satisfies both of us, honey, but I don't seem to be able to find one."

3. Express your faith in their ability to figure it out. Our adolescents look to us as mirrors reflecting our reassurance that they can handle their situation. If we show anxiety, frustration, anger, or resentment, we're not inspiring confidence in their own ability to work through the upset. Depending on the situation, a parent might say, "Look, I know you want me to fix this, but I guess I'll have to let you be mad at me. In the meantime, I really do trust that you can come up with a solution."

4. Move away without being rejecting. In preparation for the exit, make a comment that breaks the spell but still keeps you connected. The phrase "I'll go make some tea for us" is a metaphor for any nurturing statement that shows support and implies "I'm not abandoning you." It could be something like "I hope you're doing OK with this. Let's talk again in an hour and see where you are."

5. Check back in to prove that you care and are still with them. After some time has passed, we can offer some kind of nurturance such as a back rub or hot chocolate. Nonetheless, don't expect the teen to be happy and completely over it, since resentment and frustration are likely to linger. If the tornado has lost high velocity and dwindled into mere blusters, this, in itself, is a major achievement.

This five-step process pertains to a basic communication principle: In a mutually upsetting conflict, don't try to argue about the "truth." When we flood, we regress into black-white thinking. Parent thinks X and the teen Y, and there's no chance of negotiation or resolution until everyone cools off. Once the teen starts expressing extreme thoughts like "I know I'll take the ugliest school picture tomorrow," "Nobody likes me at school," or "I'll flunk the test for sure" you're in the danger zone, and the less said, the better. We nurture our overwrought teens by diffusing their emotions, and we nurture ourselves by exiting before we lose it. If meltdowns are frequent, intense, debilitating, and pervasive, without good times in between, something serious could be at hand, and families should seek a professional consultation.

Family Story: **The Burdens of Boyhood**

Boys are less inclined than girls to express their woes, but just because boys don't talk about their feelings doesn't mean that they don't have them. By the time they reach middle school, many have internalized the "boy code" (be strong, mask your feelings, never show weakness). Not only do they hide and deny the emotions percolating inside them, they often cover them with anger.

Here's a story about everything that can go wrong in one day in the life of a typical teenage boy, including frustrations, yearnings, pent-up emotions, and an inability to speak up for himself.

A groggy Henry sinks back under his covers, figuring he has plenty of time to throw on his clothes and get ready for school, when he hears his mom screaming up the stairs, "Henry, get up or you'll miss your carpool!"

Henry thinks: *That screeching voice. Why did I stay up so late last night?*

"HENRY! I'M WARNING YOU!"

Crap, I've got a math test first period. There's always stuff on it that's not in the book, and we're supposed to figure out. This sucks—Eric borrowed my calculator.

Shuffling into the hallway, Henry yells, "I'm up, Ma. I'm waiting for the bathroom."

That brat Ellie is still in the bathroom.

Henry bangs on the door, after waiting outside the door for many minutes. Ellie, his older sister, shouts that he will just have to wait until she's finished. As they argue, Mom hurries by, reminding Henry he should have gotten himself out of bed earlier.

Everybody is against me around here. How does Ellie manage to get Mom on her side every time?

Once in the bathroom, Henry tries to deal with newly erupting pimples, but his face becomes a patchwork of swollen blotches. With a wet washcloth, he tries to flatten his hair, which is sticking out like a bristle brush. Time passing, Mom yells up the stairs, "Get down here!"

Lunging down the stairs, he discovers his carpool has left without him. Ellie, however, made the ride.

She could have asked them to wait 30 seconds. So now I have to "suffer the natural consequences" of not being ready on time and ride my bike. Spare me that line. I'm going to flunk the math test for sure.

Henry pedals furiously to school, locks his bike, and sprints to class, arriving late, out of breath, and gasping for air. The math teacher hands him the test and a detention slip. Struggling, he's stuck on the part that requires a calculator. "That's unfortunate for you," the teacher says. "You need to come prepared for class." Later, in the corridor while changing classes, Henry sees Brandeth.

I feel like crap. I know I blew that test, and now Mom and Dad will be on me even more. God, there's Brandeth. She's looking at me. Maybe she's not. She's trying to look like she's not looking at me. I don't know whether that text was for real and if Brandeth really thinks I'm cute. If that note was a set-up, I'll look really lame if I start paying attention and talking to her. Whoa, what's that?

Henry trips over himself and jerks forward, books falling out of his backpack. Sweat beads break out on his upper lip as Brandeth and the girls in her posse giggle. Two of Henry's friends whack him on the back and tease him all the way to Spanish class.

I can't let them know they're getting to me. I want to go back to yesterday and start over again. I'd get up earlier and hog the bathroom so Ellie would have to go to school with smashed hair. I could kill that test. I'd walk smoothly and coolly by Brandeth. Maybe Willie would bother her, and I'd move in and shove him off. And Brandeth would sorta be crying and look at me gratefully and reach out to me.

Henry notices the Spanish teacher standing over him, "I have told you repeatedly that I will call your parents for a conference if you do not stop daydreaming in class," she says sternly. "Where is your homework? We're waiting for you."

Later, outside at lunch recess, the guys are still razzing him about his smooth move in the hall in front of Brandeth. Although Henry tries to ignore them and shoot some hoops, he is playing poorly. "Glad you're on the other team, man," Willie snarls.

I hate these guys. I'd do anything for a couple of good baskets, but the harder I try, the more I miss, and the more crap they sling me. I'm choking. I've got to get a hold of myself.

Henry body-checks Willie. Willie pushes him, and they start knocking each other around. The track coach breaks up the scuffle, talking to the boys about thinking before acting and devising alternative problem-solving strategies to violence.

What a load of bull. He's getting off on his anti-violence lecture. Willie is doing his suck-up thing with the coach so he'll think I started the whole thing, and now maybe I'll get kicked off the track team. I don't care if I do get blamed. I'm fast. They need me.

Once home, Henry retreats to his room, plugged into his iPod. He worries about what his parents are going to do when they see his math grade. He wonders whether the Spanish teacher or the coach will call his parents. He thinks about ways to find out who sent that note and whether Brandeth thinks he's hot. He fantasizes about sex with Brandeth, about Ellie flunking a class, about Willie getting expelled, and about taking the track team to the state championship. Then, his mom catches him in bed, when he has promised to mow the lawn after school.

"How could you break your promise after what happened this morning! Henry, is there something wrong?"

She is on my case every minute. She's always begging me to talk to her about my feelings, and then I get this creepy feeling all over, like I'm being suffocated. She's looking really sad because I won't talk to her. I feel lousy, but I just want to be left alone, no demands on me.

Teens like Henry can look cold and detached from the outside, yet still be flush with anxiety, yearnings, and hurt feelings, too befuddled to articulate what they're experiencing. As any parent would, Henry's mom responds to the picture in front of her—a son lying face down on his bed, plugged into his music—and can't believe he has forgotten to mow the lawn. Mom wants to figure out what's wrong, but Henry has withdrawn, unreceptive to her bid. What teen wouldn't forget a chore after a day such as his? But Henry can't begin to reach out and tell his mom of his suffering, and his mom can't be compassionate because she doesn't know what has happened.

Ashamed of showing his emotions or any weakness, Henry is unable to talk to his teachers and explain his dilemmas. Among his peers, he has to defend his pride. Boys, in particular, can be "shame phobic," meaning that they're exquisitely attuned to losing face and will do anything to avoid it, often venting their emotions through rage and outbursts. All of Henry's vulnerability comes out as aggression, as he reacts to his classmates' teasing. As much as we deplore the "indirect aggression" of girls' social patterns (gossiping, spreading rumors, excluding others), the "direct aggression" of boys, who taunt each other mercilessly, is just as harmful, especially since boys are expected to take it and be tough.

Although boys can appear to be loners, they still want relationships with parents, teachers, and friends. They just aren't always comfortable in them, and they often lack the social skills to create desired affiliations.

Henry's list of screw-ups looks dreadful: getting up late, arguing with his sister, missing the carpool, blowing a test, getting in trouble with teachers, fighting with schoolmates, and forgetting a chore. As parents, we need to reckon with our teen's lapses, but we also need to cultivate a second sense for how much is going on in their worlds. This perspective can help us moderate our judgments and focus on helping them learn from their mistakes.

Teens are tender and fragile, and we make many demands on them. When, for example, we burst in with "Good morning" and they don't reciprocate, we're all over them, but our joviality may be too much for them. The average teen is grumpy in the morning, at a low ebb in his biorhythms, and our cheerfulness may be out of sync with his spirit. The anguish that teens can experience at the mere act of getting out of bed and getting ready to face the school day can be excruciating.

Staying Connected When Your Teen Is Shutting You Out

When our teens shut us out, we work to reconnect by appreciating their complicated lives and extending the benefit of the doubt. Much depends on choosing our moments wisely.

The easiest times to be in sync with teens are when they're in bliss, soaring because they've scored a point in a game, aced a test, or feel on top of the world on a sunny day. During these good times, we capitalize on the natural camaraderie. On the opposite end of the spectrum are the hellish moments, when teens are upset or have had a disastrous day. For these darker times, it often comes down to damage control and shrewd choosing so as not to worsen the situation.

Falling in between these two opposite states is the majority of time, the messy middle, when teens have a little attitude and want us in their lives, but prefer we stay in the background unless needed. Too many parents have unrealistic expectations, believing that everything should be pleasant and friendly at all times. Hearts set on an enjoyable relationship, they're upset when their teens snub them. A key to staying connected is accepting the messy middle. If we make an overture, but they shrug us off, we need to let it go instead of feeling insulted and subsequently pursuing them. When teens give the cue that they're not in the mood to be chummy, we'd best not get in their face about it. But—a big but!—we still have to persist in giving it a shot. Try again down the road, when they're in a different mood, and you may hit that one in 10 times when they feel like talking.

Often, moms feel responsible for keeping up the connection, but dads shouldn't be let off the hook. Because dads can be less inclined to reach out and express feelings, this different twist may encourage teens to open up and share their own. Both parents can reap the benefits of interacting with teens through chores, activities, or carpools where talking can unfold naturally or the task itself can provide the connection. And don't forget the magic of touch; back rubs, foot rubs, and shoulder rubs can be ultra-nurturing gestures that build connections.

Keep in mind that "interviewing" is not connecting. Sometimes, we need to trust that our teens absorb warmth from merely being around us in an informal way—they watch TV while we make dinner—instead of quizzing them about their lives. If we discipline ourselves not to riddle them with questions, they may relax enough to speak up.

Without a doubt, it feels like a loss when our teens become less eager to be around us, and we need to be on the lookout for the true isolation and withdrawal that signals a clinical problem. With the majority of teens, though, there will still be moments of closeness. We have to "enter on their opens"— when they signal to us that they want to talk—and this is often at an inconvenient moment, like late in the evening when we're tired. Their "opens" will be less frequent than during early childhood, but if we stay alert to their cues, keeping our prying to a minimum, these moments are as good as gold.

The 'Girl Thing' and the 'Boy Thing'

It doesn't take rocket science to discern that boys and girls are different. Witness the number of gender-related parenting books on today's bookstore shelves to realize how much information is available on the strengths and vulnerabilities of each sex.

Generally speaking, boys are prone to higher levels of activity, while girls as a group will be more verbally expressive, especially of their feelings. No matter how many gender-neutral toys parents introduce, many boys devise action toys out of their sandwiches, and girls find things to tend and befriend. Experts continue to debate the relative influence of nature and nurture on these gender-typed patterns, but suffice it to say that parents' socializing patterns and expectations play a huge role in what transpires.

Much has been written about girls' "relational identities," meaning that they're extra-sensitive to relationships and how they're seen by others, sometimes to the point of losing the "strong voices" of earlier years during adolescence. If your son doesn't get invited to an overnight by one of his friends, it's not the end of the world for him, but it could feel that way for your daughter.

Boys, on the other hand, value being physically capable and strong, and are ashamed of any sign of emotional dependency or weakness. For some, the sweetness of earlier years dissolves into a façade of bravado during adolescence. If your daughter is small, clumsy, and not good at sports, it's not the end of the world for her, but it could feel that way for your son.

Although broad-stroke gender differences tend to hold up for groups of girls and groups of boys, when it comes to individuals, temperament—their inborn personality—is a more powerful predictor of behavior than gender. What does this mean? With characteristics such as motivation, cognitive abilities, or sociability, for example, there are more differences *within* groups of girls and boys than between girls and boys. We don't want to judge girls who are rowdy or boys who are tender as odd. Plenty of girls are emotional rocks who won't talk, and plenty of boys can be highly expressive and emotional. It all depends on their individual temperaments.

That said, gender stereotyping remains alive and well and thriving in America. Parents need to be acutely sensitive to the specific pressures of growing up male or female. The double bind for many girls is that they feel the pressure to conform to the perfect girl prototype—thin, nice, accommodating, always good, and never angry—while at the same time being ambitious, confident, and competitive. Boys often experience a double bind because they're supposed to be strong, manly, and stoic, while also being empathetic to others' needs and capable of expressing feelings.

The following grid reviews some of the special pressures that sons and daughters may face:

	Girls	Boys
Special pressure:	Be physically attractive, thin, and nice.	Be macho and don't show weakness or emotions.

	Girls	Boys
Specific risks:	More likely to struggle with anxiety, depression, low self-esteem, and eating disorders. May put self in subordinate relationship with males.	More likely to be diagnosed in school as learning disabled, or categorized as having an emotional disorder, ADD, or a conduct disorder. More likely to be a victim or perpetrator of violence to self or others.
Media depiction:	Emphasis on sexuality and physical appearance.	Emphasis on hypermasculinity and images of violence.

Although most teens will feel some of these pressures, smart parenting can make all the difference. Don't accept that if your daughter is only pretty, sweet, and popular, she has it all, or if your son is only smart and athletic, he's up and running. Girls need support for developing assertiveness, not just kindness and generosity, while boys need encouragement for developing empathy, not just competitiveness. More and more research has documented that down the line, teens will need a full repertoire of social and emotional skills to be successful in their work roles and marriages, not just qualities associated with their gender.[3]

What's a parent to do to counteract the traps? Occasional admiration for female beauty and male physical exploits does little harm, but these gender-typed observations need to be balanced with equally positive reactions to women who show strength and men who show sensitivity. Parents can talk openly about the plentiful stereotypes in culture and media, such as the babes on the beach and studs to the rescue.

More than style and image are at stake: Teens' health and safety ride on the extent to which they buy into sexism. A number of studies have linked "hypermasculinity" in males to tendencies toward sexual coercion and lower sanctions on sexual aggression toward females.[4]

Dangers for girls are equally astounding. Valuing one's self for sexual appeal and behavior, to the exclusion of other characteristics, is linked to eating disorders, low self-esteem, and depression. When girls look outside of themselves for comfort and direction, fixating on their looks and weight, they become targets for the dieting, tobacco, and alcohol industries, which promise them everything. The proportion of teens' purchases spent on beauty products is up 20 percent in the last year, according to a recent teen survey.[5] They are also prime customers for liposuction and cosmetic surgery.

Talking to teens goes only so far, since actions speak louder than words. If a mother promotes "speaking up with a strong voice to men" with her daughter, but silences herself with her husband, she's sending a mixed message. The same goes for a father who encourages a son to express feelings, but keeps his own emotions bottled up inside. Fathers need to model the characteristics that they hope to engender in their sons, and mothers need to do the same for their daughters.

Research on resilient children indicates that they need only one secure attachment figure to be successful, and it can be a mother, father, relative, or other caring adult. Fathers who devote themselves to parenting provide teens with some big advantages. Longitudinal studies show that sons with involved and supportive fathers have higher measures of academic and social adjustment than sons without such support.[6] Daughters who have strong connections with their fathers during adolescence become more self-reliant and academically successful.[7]

Below are tips for parents to bust gender types:

Girls

1. Try to understand fights between mothers and daughters as a teen's attempt to gain validation; realize that behind the protest "I am different from you" is a bid to be seen as unique and competent.

2. Mothers should avoid ruminating with their daughters (i.e., excessive sharing and talking about worries). Although listening and offering support to daughters is important, there should also be a focus on solving problems and coping.

3. Fathers need to be encouraged to find ways to spend positive time with their daughters in spite of awkwardness, reluctance, and either parent's preference to take the path of least resistance, and let the mothers do the parenting.

4. Avoid praising daughters (and females in general) excessively for their appearance; focus instead on other valued traits such as resilience, self-reliance, and confidence.

5. Know that girls need the same opportunities to stretch themselves and build competencies as boys, and avoid sending messages that imply that boys can be more trusted with independence than girls.

Boys

1. Promote, model, and make time to express feelings, thoughts, and values with your sons, and limit screen time and media exposure to images of violence, aggression, and degrading portrayals of women.

2. Don't make fun of sons for crying or being vulnerable; instead, make sure they know that vulnerable feelings are just as valid as assertive, angry, and bold ones.

3. Fathers need to offer nurturing and comfort to sons, not just activity-oriented time, guy talk, or parental guidance.

4. Accept your son for any rambunctious tendencies he might have, but discourage hypermasculine values while encouraging empathy.

5. Provide outlets for your son to let off steam physically and have plenty of arenas for safe risk taking (e.g., athletics, camps, challenging employment, exploring nature, leadership opportunities).

Now more than ever, it takes a village to raise children. Whether it's a coach, teacher, pastor, relative, or neighbor, different elders in teens' lives can serve as diverse role models, promoting teens' development in ways that combine valuable characteristics of both genders.

Increased parent-child conflict is one of the universal hallmarks of adolescence. As much a part of the teen years as growth spurts, voice changes, and new cognitive abilities, quarreling between parents and teens comes with the territory. Whether conflict arises out of a disagreement or a teen's bad day, it can be a vehicle for our teens to separate from us, exaggerate their "differentness," and forge their new and special selves—or it may just be a way to dump the detritus of the day.

Despite the inevitability of some family discord, the frequency, intensity, and general character of the fighting is often within a parent's control. Always keep in mind that because we're the grownups with greater wisdom, maturity, and authority, we're also the referees, responsible for fair play, rational thinking, and calling "time out" when emotions run too hot.

Arguing occurs not only when teens are upset and itching for a battle, but when parents feel as if their teens are withholding and shutting them out of their lives. Both situations require good boundaries. By staying calm, parents can have more clarity about what's going on, contain upset and negative feelings, and choose a deliberate strategy, based on what needs to be accomplished.

Though it will take many years and a lot of parental patience, teens need to learn how to express their positions and feelings as a life skill for the workplace and in relationships. Much depends on how parents conduct themselves in highly charged situations, because we are our teen's emotional role models and coaches for their future.

Difficult moments rattle parents. To steady ourselves through the tough times, we can reflect on all of our child's good qualities and the secure attachment we've forged through thoughtful, consistent, and loving parenting. We shouldn't expect to have great conversations every day to prove our deep bond to our kids. If we're more or less confident about the job we've been doing as parents, who our adolescent is, and the relative safety of his or her situation, then when we do hit a rough patch, we can trust that the connection is still there.

CHAPTER 8

When Teens Are Mean

Why Bashing Your Teen's Friends Is a Bad Move

Few parents of adolescents escape the dilemma of the undesirable friend. Into your teen's life and home comes the kid who sends your warning antennae buzzing: the underachieving slacker, the rude dude, the provocative flirt—the friend you're worried will rub off on your teen.

Small wonder that parents fret about "peer contamination," since by age 11 youngsters spend half of their waking hours with peers. What could be better than surrounding our teens with only positive role models; squeaky-clean kids good at academics and athletics? Having the right buddies seems all the more important given teens' herd behavior and natural preference for hanging out with friends instead of parents. But the sobering truth is that it's not within our power to choose our adolescents' friends.

With young children, parents can usually engineer play dates. Obviously, we can't directly choose our young children's friends, but we're in a better position to screen out undesirable influences. Early on, friends are largely about common interests: "Sam plays soccer, I play soccer, Sam and I are friends." Around ages 11–12, the whole process of who is friends with whom shifts, and parents are more or less dealt out of the picture.

Friendship choices during the teen years are wrapped into the rich and complicated process of forming an identity. Adolescents are drawn to friends not only because of common interests but also for personality traits and new affinities. Friendship choices become a mirror of a teen's own feelings, tastes, desires, and preferences. Some of these preferences (and associated friendships) are lasting, while others are temporary—tried on and later shed as part of a teen's identity search.

Social media has altered the landscape in which teens conduct their social lives. While parents often identify social media as a top complaint, teens are adamant about the ways that it enhances their friendships. Nonetheless, as with the complexity of all things social, downsides exist — the burden of social drama, keeping up with "likes," and learning about events to which teens were not invited, for example. Still, surveys indicate that the majority of surveyed teens have made new friends online, text friends daily, feel supported by reaching out in this format, and still like talking on the phone with their friends too![1]

Many parents adore their teens' friends and admire them as role models, but many will wonder about negative peer influences at some point. When "those" friends come into our teen's lives, we're inclined to weigh in with criticism and opinions, but this approach is almost always ineffective and has a fairly predictable downside. Teens react defensively to criticism of friends. They take it personally: Badmouth my friend, badmouth me. Pointing out a friend's flaws often reinforces loyalty to that friend. Parents should always mull over why their teen is drawn to a particular friend. Let's say, for example, you catch a son trying cigarettes with a boy who seems to be a risk taker and rebel. The tendency is to point the finger at the rebel as the instigator, but the more relevant question is why the son formed this friendship. Might this choice pertain to something the son needs to explore? We might as well blame the entire adolescent identity-seeking process, not just the peer, who is only one element in that process.

Also keep in mind that a parent's role isn't just to protect. A time may come when a parent needs to extricate a teen from a peer group, but jumping in too quickly may rob the teen of a valuable learning experience about who makes a good friend and who doesn't; who helps them become a better person and who brings out their worst. Experiencing a range of friendships is one way that teens figure out who they want to be, and it helps them become wiser about relationships.

In the meantime, here are some pointers for parents who have concerns about friends:

- Friendships fluctuate during adolescence; trying to influence friendship choices with opinions, advice, and judgments can backfire and is risky at best.
- If parents believe their child is settling into the wrong group, a first step is to encourage activities with other types of peers.
- Since criticizing friends rarely works, bide your time and say nothing until you have concrete proof of your suspicions and a plan (see section later in this chapter on "banning" friends).
- When mischief occurs, let teens take the lead in examining how friends had an impact on their actions. Parents can reinforce teens' insights and praise their wise deductions.
- Express your concerns carefully and respectfully: "I have seen that Jake takes risks, and I worry that you'll get in over your head."
- Although parents can't control friendship choices, they can still state whom they're willing to take on a trip or outing, though it's important to back up preferences with as little judgment as possible.

• Keep in mind that parents sometimes misjudge adolescents. A teen may have a heart of gold, but be stuck unfairly with a bad reputation.

Despite worries about our teens' social interactions, tremendous growth occurs as teens move in and out of different friendships. Through friendships, teens learn to understand others' points of view. They develop caring behavior, figuring out how to support another person, how to share, how to be responsible in a relationship, how to stay loyal, how much is reasonable to expect from others and, likewise, how much to give of one's self. Teens pick up communication skills as they consult one another in myriad situations and discover what makes for good advice and what to keep to themselves.

Through friendships, adolescents acquire a skill base of interpersonal tools they'll need for the confusing maze of future romantic and work relationships. Because most of this valuable peer interaction occurs when parents are out of earshot, we aren't always aware of the positive qualities teens gain from peers: sensitivity, compassion, and self-knowledge. Our teens could never mature in the ways we admire without a peer culture of friendships.

Family Story: **A Mom Helps Her Daughter Outwit an 'Alpha' Friend**

All children experiment with power. While some revel in it more than others, teens test their power in diverse areas: athletic competition, video gaming, academics, and in their social relationships. Social relating has its own universe of intricate dynamics, and it takes years for teens to hone the skills to navigate relationships successfully.

Observing our teens' social worlds, we tend to notice three main things: whether they have friends; how popular they are; and what their position or status is within their group of friends. Having friends—even just one or two—is undeniably important for teens' social and emotional development, but being popular isn't. Parents sometimes worry that their teens aren't popular enough, but there is no research indicating that being popular in high school takes anyone further in life.

Dynamics around a teen's status in a group can be hard for parents to read accurately, since it's always shifting. One well-publicized, negative aspect of teen social dynamics pertains to the so-called "queen bees" and "king pins." At the top of the social hierarchy, queen bees and king pins use power to stay there, sometimes coercively. Their intimidating message to others is "Fall in line, or else."

Queen bees are known for "indirect aggression"—using underhanded techniques such as exclusion, gossip, and pressure to conform to their definition of "coolness"—to keep others on their toes; king pins are typically more directly aggressive. These ringleaders consolidate their power in their posses. Teens outside the circle often get burned in their attempts to be included, trying to sit at the group's lunch table, join their conversation, or imitate their ways. Despite the fact that kids are attracted to queen bees and king pins and their power, underlings have mixed feelings, wondering if their position in the group is secure.

Some degree of power brokering exists within most groups of teens, usually far less dramatically than teen-movie stereotypes, but it can still be conniving and hurtful. Whether it's the chess-playing set, the drama club, or just a bunch of friends, groups tend to have "alphas," the teens who head up the pack. What puts alphas on top might be their looks, style, confidence, wit, assertiveness, or physical prowess.

Positioning within a group of friends doesn't necessarily involve manipulative or mean tactics, but as parents we hear more about it when it does. Within some coteries of girls, there's lots of envy, competition, and jockeying for power and position. Girls may be chumming it up one minute, and making snide remarks behind one another's backs the next. A teen girl may spend years negotiating closeness with a girl she both admires and detests.

The following is an exchange between 15-year-old Cora and her mom, Franny. A strong girl, Cora is nonetheless stinging from recent interactions with Emma, the "alpha" in her group. Although friends, Emma keeps everyone on guard with her praises and put-downs. Cora envies her style, but is intimidated by her. Other daughters might not be as direct as Cora is with her mom, but most teenage girls will leak such goings-on to their moms because of the important role peer relationships play in their emotional lives.

Franny hits pay dirt and is able to advise Cora, because her daughter is in the mood to talk and because this mom makes the right moves. Understanding that her daughter is fascinated by Emma, Mom doesn't try to convince Cora that Emma isn't worth it and she should just drop her as a friend. Like any parent with a hurt child, Franny would love to offer her two cents, but the beauty of the following interaction is in what Mom resists saying. Mom's self-control is exactly why Cora keeps talking.

Content (*what is said*)	Process (*underlying dynamics*)
Cora: Emma and Stacy went to the mall without asking me. What kind of friends are they, anyway? I hate them, but all I can do is think	*Cora is experiencing the classic social bind—wanting inclusion, feeling terribly vulnerable about exclusion, and having the mixed*

Content (what is said)	Process (underlying dynamics)
about how I want to be invited to join them.	feelings of love and hatred for complicated friends.
Mom (Franny): These kinds of binds are the worst. I know all teens go through them, but it doesn't make it any easier. What about doing something with Lizzy?	Mom tries to offer the best medicine when responding to a young teen's upset: empathy, a rational perspective, and an attempt at solving the problem.
Cora: I don't want to be with Lizzy! She's irritating. All she does is talk about her orchestra friends. She's a total nerd. Why do you always push me toward Lizzy? I want to hang out with Emma.	Moms can try their best, but when a teen needs to unload her emotion on the nearest safe and secure relationship, she'll find a way. Moreover, she has detected Mom's agenda to encourage a friendship with a nicer friend.
Mom: Look, I'm busted. Of course I like Lizzy, because she's nicer to my daughter! But I appreciate that Emma is a more exciting friend whom you enjoy being with right now. Wait, is the word "exciting?" What would you say you like the most about Emma?	Mom is clever to own up to her genuine feelings and not be defensive. Next, she takes a stab at trying to get Cora to analyze her friendships so that Cora can better understand her confused feelings.
Cora: I don't know—she's just cool. She is so confident! She puts clothes together in a way that no one else would have the guts to do, and she looks like a model. And when she makes fun of people, she gets away with it. Stacy totally laughs along with it, even when she is the one getting picked on.	Mom struck gold in terms of engaging Cora in a thinking process instead of just an emotive process of dumping on Mom. Cora is drawn to Emma's social traits, which give her power—style, confidence, and savvy with peers.

Content *(what is said)*	Process *(underlying dynamics)*
Mom: It sounds like despite the put-downs, Emma has a knack for having people enjoy the sparks of being around her.	*Mom walks a thin line here of "active listening," where she acknowledges the positive aspects of being around a mean girl, but also manages to slip in a reference to Emma's indirect aggression.*
Cora: Yeah, it's really fun to be with Emma, until it's your turn to get a jab—like when she made fun of my "adorable baby fat" in front of everyone. I wanted to kill her.	*Cora's remarks reflect the mixed bag of hanging out with alpha girls. They have skills for making fun and slinging velvet daggers at the same time.*
Mom: You could laugh and turn it around with a compliment like "I only wish that I could have a perfect body like yours." But you'll need to say it like you mean it, without sarcasm, or it could bite you back.	*Mom restrains herself from condemning Emma, knowing that Cora would cut her off and defend her friend. Instead, she offers an effective ploy—the disarming compliment.*
Cora: That would be a good one, because she's always talking about how her legs are too short and her hair is too frizzy And, I get it . . . I'd show her she isn't getting to me.	*Cora has already indicated that she is bugged by the way Stacy tolerates Emma's put-downs, so she is relieved to imagine alternatives.*
Mom: Yeah, well, it might at least give her pause because "perfect" is rare when it comes to bodies. It's a way to stand up to her and it doesn't involve handing back a put-down, which could really be risky with someone like her.	*Mom knows that confronting someone as powerful as Emma should be saved for dire necessity, since it can cause big dramas when girls are forced to take sides. Plus, Cora could end up exiled, and she has already revealed that she wants to keep this "friend"—at least for the time being.*

Skirmishes like Cora and Emma's typify teen girl social relating. Like many top dogs, Emma is facile and has a mean streak. Confronting them with their meanness or returning the insult could be disastrous, because they know how to stay one-up and make others look like idiots. Mom wisely refrains from demonizing Emma, realizing that this is not a simple case of dropping the girlfriend. Instead, she suggests a way for Cora to deflect the put-down. Cora may not use her mom's suggested retort; together, they might try coming up with other options. One would be to use a one-liner that shows she's "Teflon," such as, "Yeah, I guess my baby fat is adorable," or "Yeah, I feel lucky when I watch music videos—curvy is definitely in." The point is not necessarily to supply teens with the exact words, but with the right attitude and alternatives to just laughing along.

Instead of focusing on Emma as a bad person, Mom stimulates her daughter's thinking about options. A major goal when your teen has a mean friend is to keep the channels of communication open. This allows Cora to express negative feelings about how she is being treated; later, she can decide whether to keep trying to stay close to Emma. After all, the friendship is Cora's decision, and she does seem to be coping fairly well, critiquing the pros and cons of this friendship.

How Parents Can Blow It by Overreacting to Peers

Cora's mom is a realist who understands that "girl stuff" is best coached from the sidelines. Instead of overreacting to Cora's emotions, she appreciates her mixed feelings about Emma. Also, Mom doesn't moralize about virtues. When Cora lashes out, describing Lizzy as a nerd, Franny refrains from getting on a soap box about being a good friend. All teens struggle with the "coolness" factor and may put others down to keep themselves up.

Some parents overreact when their teen is hurt by a mean friend. Failing to grasp the complicated universe of teen social interaction, they may view their own child as the good kid and the other as bad. Although the following patterns often arise instinctively, they have distinct downsides and are to be avoided.

Mother bears go on the attack to protect their young and eliminate the threat. Particularly in middle schools, girls vie for position and power in ways that can seem threatening. Because Franny slows down and listens to Cora, she knows what she's working with. Like most alpha girls, Emma has traits that are intriguing, ones that Cora is trying to figure out for herself. And keep in mind: Bashing your teen's friends is bashing your own teen.

Rescuers also want to protect, but they move in, take over, and solve the problem, trying to spare their teen any distress or hurt. Although Franny makes one attempt to suggest that Cora hang out with a nice friend, she self-corrects and drops this social bandage. Instead, she engages Cora in her own exploration of what attracts her to Emma.

Direct busters are straight-shooters who advise with oversimplified responses like "Just tell her off." Given normal group dynamics with girls, straightforward talk rarely works successfully with alpha girls.

A direct buster might suggest that Cora say to Emma, "Talking about my baby fat hurts my feelings," or "You are mean to talk about my baby fat." Alpha girls like Emma are clever, using tactics that can be denied. Emma could reply, "But Cora, I said it was adorable!" or "But Cora, you are so sensitive! Can't you take a joke?" Then Cora would be left with more egg on her face.

Advising teens to express their hurt feelings is a dubious recommendation. A good rule is to express vulnerable feelings when there's reason to believe the person hurting them may respond empathetically. Mixed-message teasing requires deft retorts that throw the teaser off balance and make it less fun.

Victim reinforcers engage in too much talking and commiserating. Although empathizing with a hurt teen can be a real gift, going overboard with this well-intended gesture puts too much focus on your child as victim and may reinforce this role.

Some parents engage in "dumpster diving," digging around for dirt on friends as a way of connecting with their teen. Teens learn to bring their garbage to parents to gain sympathy and attention. Catered to in this way, teens never develop skills to cope with the slings and arrows of normal adolescence. A better move is to encourage coping responses; one technique is to recall an episode when a teen successfully managed a crisis and remind her of what she did in that circumstance.

Mother bears, rescuers, direct busters, and victim reinforcers share the same disadvantage: Trying to be a caring and involved parent, they fail to arm their teens with the strength and resilience they need to rebuff inevitable social nastiness. Doing too much sends the message "You can't do it," and thus children learn they are helpless or incompetent. Over time, some kids find power in letting others do for them instead of relying on themselves. A parent's job is not to sanitize, purge, or remove social problems. Parents support, guide, and challenge teens to manage their own problems and out of that experience, teens become more skilled, competent, and empowered in the ways of the world.

Adolescent Social Bruises

Social bruises are as normal for adolescents as skinned knees are for preschoolers. As parents, we naturally hear more about the "sins of others" than our own teen's offenses, especially with daughters who express vulnerable feelings more openly. It can come as a surprise to learn that your teen isn't just receiving insult and injury; she's also dishing them out. Knowing this can help us maintain perspective and be less reactive to our teen's social bruises, upsetting though they may be.

Although a few go unscathed, most teenagers will occasionally:
- Have a significant quarrel with a friend. Sometimes they will start it, and sometimes the friend will.
- Be dropped by a friend (same sex or otherwise)—and most of them will drop someone else.
- Be on the receiving end of a hurtful comment or action such as a mean or nasty post—and most will say or do something hurtful to someone else.
- Be the object of gossip—and most will gossip about others.
- Be excluded in some way from a group they want to belong to or a party they want to attend—and most will conspire to do the same to another.
- Lose an important friend over a misunderstanding that is never cleared up.
- Feel social pressure to do something they normally wouldn't do—and most will pressure another to do the same.
- Be unable to share a grievance openly with a friend—and most will be blind to something in their behavior that a friend should tell them about but doesn't.
- Be overly critical of a friend—and most will be defensive about or hurt by receiving criticism that is unfairly harsh.

During elementary school, we could directly influence whether our children did the "right" thing, making sure Valentines were distributed to everyone, being discreet about who received birthday-party invitations, and prompting our children to say they're sorry. By middle school, we're no longer in that position. Still, depending on the bruise's severity, we have options for responding.

The following are four choices for parents when they realize it's their teen that's being mean.

Ignore it and let it play itself out. Example: Your teen doesn't want to invite an old friend to a birthday party. With mild forms of inclusion or exclusion, it's legitimate to see these decisions as the teen's prerogative, despite the fact that there may be hurt feelings. Often, repercussions occur, and teens can learn from these natural consequences.

Use the Socratic method, asking questions to stimulate thinking without weighing in. Example: You hear from a friend that your son hurt a peer's feelings with mild teasing. Instead of insisting on a direct apology, you could ask, "Regardless of whether you think he was too sensitive and should not have told his mother, what might be some ways to remedy this situation?" "Is it ever right to apologize for hurt feelings, even if you think you did nothing wrong?" "Say we're not talking about you here. What might someone you really respect do in this situation?" Teens may detect their parents' motive and shut down. Still, the questions may sink in and provoke thought.

Take a position, but let them choose. Example: Your teen fudges a lame excuse for getting out of a commitment with one friend to take another up on a much better offer. Obviously, you tell him you disapprove of this dishonesty. Although you tell him exactly where you stand, you leave it up to him to decide one way or another. You let him incur the negative results of his decision, including the guilt.

Step in and get involved. Example: Your teen spreads a lie through gossip, and you learn about it. With this kind of offense, you take direct action of some kind. More often than not, a teen will deny it or weave a convoluted story to cover her tracks, but even then, your harsh judgment, rebuke, and whatever steps you decide to take will make an impression, even if she doesn't confess.

For most social bruises, as long as we are able to provide oversight, guidance, and support as needed, it is almost always preferable to let adolescents resolve their own issues. How tempting it is to directly intercede! But the reality is that adolescents will wrong and hurt others socially, and be wronged and hurt themselves, and therein resides their platform for social learning.

Nevertheless, it's critical for parents to stay watchful so that if a social bruise becomes a true injury we can shift into an intervening mode and get teens the help they need. A lot of initially benign social stinging can get out of hand and escalate into deeply harmful behavior. Having our eyes open for injury with stoic kids is especially important, since they tend to "suck it up"—not complain or ask for help, even when being victimized.

Social Cruelty on a Spectrum

Except for a small percentage of sweet, gentle, or naïve teens, nearly all will instigate social slights at some point in their shifting patterns of friendships. Chalk it up to the fray of youth—the hormones, competitiveness, developing brain, insensitivity, and impulsivity. With put-downs, rumors, gossip, and teasing, parental responses should be on par with the injury.

True cruelty exists on a spectrum, from mild to moderate to malicious. We don't want to confuse classic mean-girl moves such as gossiping behind someone's back or mild teasing with the malicious bully-victim dynamic. More extreme, "bullying" is a term used to describe the regular and purposeful tormenting of a victim.

A key feature of all gradations of bullying is that it happens repeatedly. Examples would be relentless spreading of lies on the Internet, a pattern of overt sexual harassment, or making someone the brunt of a mean prank, such as a group of kids ganging up and swiping someone's stuff off the athletic field every day.

The old advice to "just ignore" bullies doesn't work, because bullies have an instinct for when someone is trying to steer clear and will not be deterred. Like piranha sensing blood, they can really go for it. Some schools have a bully culture, and in this case parents will want to make sure administrators and teachers are acting decisively to counteract it. Since some teens who are being bullied clam up, behavioral symptoms such as declining grades, wanting to avoid school and social events, and changing moods may be the only clues. If your teen is being victimized, report it to the school and consult a professional, since this is serious business requiring intervention.

With occasional mild to moderate meanness, parents' responses are less clear-cut and usually involve careful delving into the problem and making judgment calls. One nasty incident doesn't imply bullying, and even something that looks bad can involve extenuating circumstances that fit into a larger story.

Let's say a pack of rowdy boys eggs your son's bedroom window. With a little investigation, you might discover that your own son has made similar mischief. Parents' responses always need to take into account whether their own teen may have played into the act. Another example might be if a boy in your daughter's class posts a remark about her "perky boobs" on Instagram. When confronted, it may turn out to be a stupid, impetuous first offense by a naïve, apologetic boy. Consequences will be doled out for the boy, but parents should avoid focusing on the daughter's victimization.

Interestingly, researchers have noted an increase in teen online harassment over the last decade, largely because of the rise in girls' online aggression and cruelty—i.e. sending or posting comments by others online.[2]

Another situation calling for careful judgment is when your teen is a bystander, watching something ugly but not instigating the incident. Teens are in this bind more than parents realize. It takes a lot of courage for bystanders to step off the sidelines and discourage meanness, especially if the perpetrator is popular and your teen wants to curry favor with him. Don't be surprised if your teen sides with the powerful kid.

Instead of just scoffing, "Boys will be boys" or "Girls will be girls," parents have the option of choosing this battle and talking to their teen about the situation. Even if your teen feels that she can't take on the powerful teen directly, you can encourage her to distract the perpetrator, perhaps with a witty remark, or by making a move that subtly counteracts the cruelty. Suggest that she enlist some friends to help and encourage her to strengthen her "upstander" skills in safe but direct ways.

How 'In' a Teen's World Should You Be?

Parents tend to have a whole set of opinions about when, where, and how to be involved in their teen's lives. For the most part, our parenting biases and inclinations are based on our personalities (anxious, rigid, or extroverted, for example), our own childhood experiences, personal histories with friends, values, perceptions of our teen's social situation, and parenting philosophies. Out of all this emerges a wide range of different approaches to parenting teens, from parents who think that all Internet activity should be monitored to those who would never even consider it; from parents so anxious that they routinely give their teen the third degree to those who assume that if they don't stumble upon social mischief, it isn't happening.

Whether your tendency is to be hypervigilant or hands off, a good guideline for degree of parental involvement is your teen's track record. If a sophomore in high school has been in trouble regularly with his push-the-envelope personality and big appetite for thrill seeking, his parent will want to watch him like a hawk in risky situations, such as when he and his friends start driving—and maybe postpone his getting a driver's license! On the other hand, if your son and his friends always follow the rules, and thus far there has hardly been a bump, surveillance of his every move would be overkill.

Most teens are neither big-time risk takers nor models of perfect self-discipline. Parents of most teens stand a middle ground and:

- Stay observant.

- Remain on call and available.
- Insist on the "Big Five" (knowing where their teens are; who they're with; when they're coming home; transportation details; and contact information and agreements).
- Stay apprised of social events and transactions.

These areas usually give parents enough information to determine whether or not they need to move in and monitor more closely. If your teen is managing his social life well and you have no reason to believe otherwise, a good default position for you is to support your teen's social independence—meaning that you don't need to investigate any further than the list given above.

Beyond your own observations, here are other sources of information to consider when determining how much to be "in" or "out" of your teen's social world:

- **Your friends and peers.** Do they tell you that you are overprotective or over-involved? Have they told you that you might be asleep at the wheel? Friends or peer parents can be apt judges because they know you and your teen.

- **Teachers or school counselors.** Experts on teens, they also observe your teen in a different setting. If teachers tell you about problems between your teen and peers, consider following their recommendations.

- **Your child.** Obviously, teens can have a conflict of interest when they request more social independence, but they can also be justified when they tell a parent asking a zillion personal questions that they are crossing a line. If you suspect your teen's complaint has merit, circle back and consult with trusted friends, family members, or school staff.

- **Spot checks.** Even if a teen's social life is running fairly smoothly, parents may want to check up occasionally on their whereabouts and whether they're following house rules on Internet and cell-phone use. Talking with other parents on a casual basis can yield new insights. For older teens, wait up now and then for them to come home.

- **Your nose.** Parents routinely find out important information when they follow up on "parent intuition" and get a whiff of something amiss. To detect subtle cues, parents need to be involved enough to pick up on the signals.

Strategic Moves for Banning Friends

Mama-bear and papa-bear reactions come only too naturally whenever we sense a bad influence on our precious cubs. Given our fiercely protective instincts, we need to think through our moves carefully before intervening to banish the "bad" friend.

Let's say, for example, your son acts very disrespectfully when he's around a friend named Joe; or you've heard that Joe uses marijuana; or Joe has failing grades; or Joe dresses in a "gangster" style (according to you). Any of these reasons are sufficient cause for raised parental antennae, but they aren't reasons to banish Joe—at least not yet. Instead, you engage in a thoughtful process that extends the benefit of the doubt and establishes solid evidence.

Here are your moves:

Don't tip your hand about Joe. The most important thing is to be wise about what you say, keeping your mouth shut and steering clear of character assassination. If you criticize Joe, not only will your son defend Joe, he may be even more attracted to him. Also, he'll be less likely to share information about Joe, becoming more secretive and perhaps even lying.

Put your son on notice with careful conversations. Be clear with your son that you're concerned about his new behaviors, whether it's increased sassiness or sloppiness about punctuality, kitchen messes, or video-game limits. Despite the fact that these behaviors surfaced when Joe arrived on the scene, you focus on your son's need to clean up his act. Be very strict about compliance with the Big Five, and when your son tells you that you're a control freak, reply indifferently that you're merely doing your job.

Be more vigilant about monitoring. Use all your senses to detect evidence of foul play. Check his pockets when doing the laundry and do a "spot check" when you happen to be looking for something in his closet. Check digital correspondence more actively, in keeping with whatever contract you have in place. Take care not to violate the contract yourself, unless you have reason to believe your teen already has, and then tell him first.

Weigh the costs and benefits of violating privacy. With no evidence of illegal activity, poking into diaries, email, and backpacks is risky. Run an analysis to decide whether to take this step. The cost may be that your teen finds out, blows up, and your relationship takes a hit. The benefit might be discovering crucial information about drug use or other risky business. Teens consider these moves violations of their rights and of trust, so take care before crossing these boundaries. However, your nose is your nose. Respect that, too!

Use logic like a court of law. If you discover concrete evidence that Joe and your son are implicated in an illegal activity (shoplifted merchandise, drugs or drug paraphernalia, empty beer bottles) or there just may have been too many family-rule violations, you can make a judgment to ban Joe—for period of time that fits the crime. For mild infractions, your son and Joe "take a break" for a couple of weeks. After a hiatus, they can try socializing again, but only if your son's conduct has been without blemish.

The key is to stay objective and fact-based: "You came in late three times, continue to be disrespectful in his company despite warnings, and didn't respond to my texts or calls on several occasions. You two don't bring out the best in one another. You may have regular privileges with other friends, but we're taking a break from social rights to Joe for a month. If your conduct is excellent and you haven't fudged on this restriction, in a month, we'll reconsider access to Joe."

Even if guilty as charged, this will be bad news for your son, who is likely to throw a fit to resist the ban. Your effectiveness depends on staying calm and succinct, and using your thinking brain instead of the emotional one— the one that wants to spill your fears and valid concerns about Joe's influence. Then leave the room; go do something, so that your frustrated and angry son doesn't cut off his nose to spite his face by cussing you out—because then you'll have to deal with that, too!

Nudging Shy Teens Along the Social Path

Parents of teens with big social appetites and "iffy" friendships have extra parenting work to rein in their bucking broncos and monitor their relationships. Likewise, parents of shy kids have extra parenting work to engineer social opportunities that expand the teen's narrow comfort zones. In either situation, parents need to accept their teens' inborn temperaments and deal with these challenges in positive ways that avoid damaging the teen's self-image.

The United States is a tough place to be a shy person, for we celebrate the go-getters. Although the "emotional intelligence" movement has challenged our country's myopic love affair with IQ, a new generation of parents fears that its children will not be successful unless they're social giants. Concerns about shy teens abound: Will my teen's self-esteem plummet without a group of friends? Will he develop the necessary social skills? How can I help my child expand her world when she's fighting me every step of the way?

Although shyness and introversion are related, there are important distinctions. Introverts prefer solitary pursuits to social ones, but they don't fear social contact as do shy individuals. A common problem for parents of both shy and introverted teens is the teen's willful refusal to initiate social outings or participate in activities. Fighting can ensue, as parents promote socializing and the child resists. Shy teens are more hysterical as they dig in their heels than introverts because their refusal is based on anxiety and genuine feelings of dread. By their child's adolescence, parents are turning themselves into pretzels trying to find friends or activities the child is willing to accept, while teens persist in their resistance.

This is exactly what had happened with 14-year-old Shen, a shy teen, and her parents, who were extroverts by nature. Although Shen enjoyed the friendship of an older girl next door and did well at school, she threw a tantrum when her mother tried to arrange social plans. She fought with her parents about trying anything new, boycotting sports and play dates, dropping out of extracurricular activities, and not showing up at birthday parties. Shen's parents had reached the end of their rope. The problem with their approach was that they pushed, when nudging and accepting would have been a better strategy.

With shy teens, the first step is for parents to deal with their own anxiety. If Shen doesn't feel accepted for who she is, her anxiety about everything will be intensified. No matter how immensely parents love their children, when they're anxious about their child's temperament, it transmits messages that say, "We wish you were different."

Shen's parents needed to overhaul their approach. Shy teens have the toughest time in groups of peers. When parents ask them if they want to invite friends somewhere, it's like asking someone who is afraid of drowning to jump into the deep end. The social stimulus is too overwhelming for anxious kids. A first step is to start with much less threatening social engaging—maybe working with animals, preschoolers, the disabled, or the elderly. From these options, Shen agreed to volunteer two days a week at a nursing home, as long as her mom went with her the first few times.

Here are some recommendations for helping shy teens:
- Avoid referring to your child's shyness. Labels contribute to solidifying this self-image.
- Focus on building her strengths as you would with any child's profile of strengths and weaknesses. If she loves volunteering at the animal shelter, she might next expand to a dog-walking business.
- Don't confuse popularity with friendships. If your child has a couple of

peers she considers friends and doesn't complain of loneliness, then back off on big efforts to promote sociability.

• Trust that your teen is developing socially if he is in social settings of any kind—school, extended family gatherings, or any activity outside the home.

• Model social skills and bring your child along, allowing her to "piggy back" on your own social opportunities.

• Use sweeteners, such as tickets to a fun outing, to encourage your teen to invite a friend along. Even if the teen is more of a spectator than a participant, it still counts because he's out in a public setting.

• Keep trying new endeavors, and package the proposals as a matter of family values, not an assessment of the child's deficiencies. Whether it's attending the youth group at the family's place of worship or packing rice bags at the neighborhood food bank, such acts promote the value that life isn't "all about me," while also enhancing social skills and cultural exposure.

Helping shy teens means working both sides of the equation, accepting small steps, while also continuing to nudge (not push!) along the social path. As a general rule, parents should allow teens some leeway to select the setting based on their comfort zone. Teens get to choose where, but not whether, they go. Encourage small steps toward goals, and even if the teen relates very little to others in her chosen role, it's a great beginning.

Parents sometimes become invested in a fairy-tale vision of their teens' social lives, hoping for all the right friends, right social interactions, and right activities. In reality, because they're on a steep learning curve, teens struggle through many imperfect situations with friends. They feel pressures to play the social game and conform to rules about what's cool and what isn't. It's tough either way: Act too much outside of the lines, and you're not included, but too much inside the lines with too much conforming, and you don't develop as an individual.

Because teen social culture has intricacies beyond a parent's grasp, we can trot in too quickly with our solutions, offering simplistic, unrealistic advice. Staying watchful and providing oversight is critical, but a parent's role in a teen's social life often boils down to a set of guidelines: Don't bash their friends; stimulate their thinking about their situation; support them in their problems, but allow them to have the experience of resolving their own difficulties. Out of the untidy process of problem solving, struggling, and dealing with the consequences of their actions, teens become wiser about relationships. As long as teens aren't overwhelmed, we should support their independence.

For all of our concerns about peers, we should also appreciate how much they give to our teens. Peers affirm each other, laughing at jokes, pinging off each other's ideas, and offering heartfelt advice.

CHAPTER 9

When Screen Time Dominates Your Teen's Life

For all of the dangers, abuses, and distractions of today's wired world, the upsides are unprecedented:

- A young violinist in a rural area eager to improve his skills can view recordings of performances by Toscanini on YouTube.
- A teen boy who is gay and feeling depressed can enter an educational chat room on gender identity and read information that makes him feel life is worth living.
- A disorganized middle-schooler can keep track of homework assignments through an interactive Web site with his teacher and receive quick answers to questions.

At one time, the Web was likened to the Wild West, with no one in charge, outlaws lurking around every bend, and massive freedom to roam and run into trouble. More than a region, it's a vast universe where the orbits and galaxies of digital travel invite endless exploration.

Media plays an extraordinary role in the lives of tweens and teens, as they effortlessly juggle a circus of media connectivity. Millennials (Gen Y, who came of age around the turn of the century and grew up with the Web) have been described as the digital generation. Fully embedded in all things digital, post-millennials (Gen Z, reaching maturity after 2007, the year the iphone was introduced) have been dubbed both iGen and Generation Media. In 2010, U.S. teens spent an average of 8.5 hours a day interacting with digital devices, up from 6.5 hours in 2006.[1] This astonishing statistic and the trajectory it suggests is worth contemplating, to consider all the things teens aren't doing and learning—and likewise, are doing and learning — as they interact with screens.

Having the latest gadgets is a rite of passage for today's teens. Different generations have always had something to make them feel "adult," whether it was getting a first pair of knickers, having a first drink, or receiving a first kiss. Rites of passage have accelerated, and even very young children know how to tap into the digital world, where they can to learn how to mimic behaviors of teen culture to feel older.

By preadolescence, most kids are thoroughly adept with touchscreens and devices. The powerful genie is already out of the bottle and possibilities are expansive. There is no one-size-fits-all approach for parents regarding media use in the family, but one website, commonsensemedia.org, can supply parents with parent-child contracts, up to date research and reasonable guidance that parents can trust.[2] This website serves as a clearinghouse of information that virtually all health practitioners and experts use as their North Star. Key points for parents to consider are agreements about content access, screen time limits, and rules about how the medium is used; for example, the digital transmission of content and postings.

Teens consider having a cell phone as a basic right and probably already have one by the time parents are reading this book. Although many parents believe they are enhancing their kids' safety by purchasing them one, cells are more about convenience and allowing your tween or teen access to the digital spectrum shared by their peers. If your child doesn't yet have a cell, consider holding off until it's really necessary—and "necessary" could be because your teen is excluded by being the only one without one among her friends. Nonetheless, cells usually wind up being another time-waster — something to monitor and manage. Along with use comes the potential for abuse, when, for example, teens lie about their whereabouts. Even with GPS, parents need to be aware of teen scams in which friends hold phones for one another to send out a location signal of where they are supposed to be, even though they are not. Acquiring their first cell, tweens and young teens—especially social ones who plead persistently for them—will almost always go overboard, interacting with their devices at every opportunity to look and feel important, and then, of course, losing them. Before you sign a contract with a service provider, get your own written agreement ready with your teen, with consequences for misuse spelled out.

Parents can be dazzled as their teens teach themselves computer coding, send texts from phones within their pockets, or whip off new lingo. Unable to keep up, many parents give up trying to control technology before they even get started, despite the fact that "giving up" is one thing experts say you shouldn't do.

It's standard knowledge that teens are online with people, places, and things that are unknown to parents. We wouldn't give our teens free rein in their social worlds, but the majority of parents leave their children unchaperoned in the world of the Web. In the same way that we impose limits, allowing teens to go to a dance, but not an unsupervised party, parents need to create guidelines for cyberspace. To get started, parents can work out a "learner's permit" that begins very conservatively and then allows more freedom as teens gain experience and show they can control themselves on this supercharged information superhighway. Once teens establish a track record of responsible use, parents don't need to be checking over shoulders as much.

Out of these circumstances emerge these recommendations for parents:

1. Do your best to become cybersavvy, because your kids already are! You won't know what your kids are up to unless you're informed of the possibilities. One good technique is to have your teen show you how things work.

2. Although teens crave the latest gadgets, consider stalling before handing technology over to them. Nevertheless, talk about it early in elementary school, because even third-graders can be egged on by older kids to forward illicit material without knowing what they're doing.

3. Be an authoritative parent, characterized by warmth and support, structure and supervision, and effective communication strategies. Although you can't control the Internet, you can create and enforce rules for how teens use their time, according to your values. Teens who are out in the world, involved in a range of healthful activities, will naturally have less time to spend with media. Research indicates that parental permissiveness plays a role in excessive media use, but the effectiveness of parental control is less clear. A couple of studies cite a correlation between authoritarianism and less media use, but experts caution against too much control because teens find workarounds.

4. Be proactive and set policies before teens get in over their heads. Once kids are old enough to use technology independently, usually by fifth grade, establish guidelines. Because fifth-graders will still listen to parents, the timing is right to develop good habits.

5. Policies about digital games, cells, and other media work similarly to social and physical freedom to roam. The more competence, trustworthiness, and good habits displayed, the more parents grant independence. When infractions or difficulties occur—homework suffering or isolating from real-world social engagement, for example—more stringent rules or temporary pullbacks can be imposed. Almost all parents need to tweak their media use policies at some point. It should be a "living document," updated and adjusted in the interest of instilling healthy media consumption.

6. Parents can assume the role of digital mentor. Instead of shaming children for their media use, parents can support and guide children on how to use media appropriately, learning and building skills to thrive in the digital world.[3] Increasingly, media experts are noting that parents need to set a good example themselves, since they are often more fused to their screen than their kids!

The tips and guidelines below will be pertinent to conversations you'll have with your kids throughout middle and high school. They can also lay the groundwork for a "graduated-use permit," starting in about fifth grade and can be supplemented with others found on commonsensemedia.org:

- Keep computers in communal family spaces, allowing parents to cast an eye on the screen occasionally. Reserve laptops in rooms for older, mature teens.
- Remind teens never to share their passwords or any personal information (name, birth date, address, school, age, gender) with anyone they meet on the Web.
- Be emphatic about never meeting anybody in person whom teens have met online, and make it clear that people give false information all the time.
- For social networking sites, know the friend lists for young teens. Also have your child's passwords so you can do spot checks. Anything posted on the Net is public, and therefore not a violation of their privacy.
- Particularly with middle-schoolers, risk-taking teens, or teens with shaky bearings, do an occasional spot check on online activity and ask to see their profile page on social network sites "tomorrow," giving them a chance to clean it up.
- Establish limits and rules for when they can be online and where they can and cannot go. Restrict use when the agreement is violated.
- Post notes: "Never put anything in print that you don't want others to see."
- Talk about the potential downside of acting on impulse: Fun now, disaster later. Teens can have a great old time being included in social media postings, commenting, and text forwarding and lose sight of trouble in the making when they help spread rumors.
- Remind teens, "What you post online stays in cyberspace forever." Nothing is private and anything can be tracked back by future employers and others.
- Use filters and outlaw pornographic and other questionable Web sites according to your values.

- If parents have information that technology use is a problem for their children, supervise it more closely and yank it temporarily if need be.
- Remove cells and laptops at bedtime. Consider sticking everyone's gadgets in a closet in your room for recharging. The research is clear as a bell on the importance of sleep for teens and their need for at least nine hours a night. If their cell is in their bed with them, it will be used, and each little ding means sleep disruption and the loss of the sacred sleep architecture equated with mental health and optimal cognitive functioning.

As with cars and inexperienced teen drivers, the whole point is to make sure teens know how to use technology safely through authoritative parenting policies. And, as they would with a teen's social life, parents should observe the delicate balance of knowing when to step in. The more risk-taking and sensation-seeking the teen, the more vigilant parents will need to be. Kids who push the envelope, are impulsive, and like to show off are as likely to do something dumb online as they are in other social situations—maybe even more so, given the pace of interacting.

Supervise middle-schoolers closely, since they don't always grasp the consequences of their impetuous actions. Much of the lure of social media for them relates to their developmental surge. Unsure of themselves, they feel nervous if they're not in touch with friends and processing daily events online with them—just as teens used to do on landlines. It's as if they think, "I'm online, therefore I'm connected, I belong, and I matter."

Online socializing tends to peak in eighth or ninth grade and then drop off somewhat. Even if they elect not to get their driver's licenses, older teens are able to move about more independently to be with friends. Their social worlds expanding, many prefer to meet up with friends in real life. They become surer of themselves as they mature and seek more authentic relationships, preferring "face time" rather than "virtual time" with peers.

Family Story: **A Turbo-Charged Identity**

Something is amiss with 13-year-old Pilar. Not only is she unusually tired and moody, her grades are declining. Also, there's the matter of her screen fixation, a source of contention in the family. Pilar's parents have made sure she has an assortment of school and community extracurricular activities that keep her active but not overly scheduled. They've followed the guidelines of restricting computer use to a family space and, likewise, have had many discussions about her screen use. In reality, however, they are constantly arguing about it, and her on-the-go parents struggle to monitor limits.

One night, her dad awakens at 2 a.m. His sixth sense tells him that something is up in the household. Is Pilar sneaking out to meet friends, he wonders? Instead, he finds his daughter absorbed in a different kind of drama — a secret social media account for teen bloggers with videos and photos. Pilar's blog created under the identity, "Photo Diva," is a dramatized, highly embellished version of herself. Not only is Pilar famous among her peers, she is also under so much pressure to keep her growing readership entertained that she has resorted to midnight computer rendezvousing.

Pilar's blog features saucy photographs of schoolmates, vamping before the camera, accompanied by witty stories, all fictional, elaborate, and very clever. Letting her schoolwork slide, she is devoting enormous time and energy to get kids to pose for her, usually doing something slightly risqué or embarrassing, for her daily entries.

Tweens and teens have always yearned to perfect their image, belong to the cool tribe, and manage impressions others have of them as they run, not walk, into the social world of adolescence. Now, instead of meeting others and making impressions in the physical world, they can curate the desired look according to their own whims, 24/7 online, using countless social media sites. Teens can take scores of selfies, edit out their pudgy imperfections and post them daily, looking wildly attractive, popular and happy all the time. Even though kids know that fakeness abounds in this curation process, they may still feel lousy because the images generate a feeling that everyone else's life is better than theirs. The explosion of "YouTube" fame, where a teen can be known to thousands overnight, feeds into more and more teens wanting to seek importance and fame for themselves. Absorbing messages from the media, teens today view fame as a future goal and aspiration.[4]

Infuriated, Pilar's parents can't believe she has deliberately disobeyed the family policy—and for such a purpose! For all of their efforts to round out their daughter's interests, they're appalled that she has duped them, turning away from her many talents and "real" self to focus on a bogus online identity. "That's it! You've broken the rules too many times, and we're tired of fighting about it," the parents announce. "We're pulling the plug on your technology. No more Photo Diva!"

Pilar goes ballistic. "You can't do this to me! This is my whole social life! Everyone reads my blog—I have 1430 followers! You don't know what you'd be doing to me! If you think my grades have gone down now, just wait."

Pilar's parents know this is a dramatic overreaction, but they also wonder whether their own response is similarly extreme.

A Calm Approach: As serious as Pilar's flagrant violation of family policy is, her parents are also rightly concerned about her identity development. When teens spend more time networking online than in face-to-face situations, how do they know who they are or when they are truly accepted for themselves?

But Pilar has a point: Taking away her computer completely for an indefinite period of time is cutting her off from peers. Cyberspace is their mall times a hundred. After putting in a full day with school and other activities, Pilar's most efficient way to socialize is online. What she is doing is deceptive, but producing Photo Diva has a creative side. Blogs are the perfect vehicle for dramatic self-expression, especially for highly verbal girls. To date, teen girls are some of the most prolific content creators on the Web.

Pilar's parents will need to address her lying, the sexualized nature of her identity curation, the use of friends' images without permission, and the potential for exploitation. As a consequence of breaking the rules, she should have some time off from the computer. Similar to a teen fender-bender, parents take away the car for a while, but let them back behind the wheel with greater monitoring. Pilar has been out drag racing online, but in today's wired world, it's more logical to impose a break, then let her back on with supervision for an hour a day and then two. Her parents might also consider regular checking of her Internet "travel history," since they now know that she likes to roam secretly.

With this kind of incident, parents will need to work within the limitations of their daughter's 13-year-old brain. Pilar won't be able to understand the full implications of how her online flights of fancy could be undermining her identity development and her social-skill development, particularly since this feels like her "whole social life."

Pilar's blog is a lot for a 13-year-old girl to sustain. If teens are at school, involved in activities, doing homework, and having family dinners, there won't be much time left over to become addicted to social networking. Now that Pilar's parents are aware of her rule breaking, they can redouble their efforts to enforce their limits on social media. She can still enjoy a toned-down version of her Photo Diva persona, but only as one aspect of her identity. Her parents can insist that blogging be linked to an agreement to engage also in real-world endeavors, be it as a staff member of the yearbook, jazz dancer, or volunteer at a soup kitchen.

Only too easily can teens get wrapped up in a giant online popularity contest and an obsessive and competitive pursuit of "likes" on Instagram and other social media sites. Even though they know that much of this process is fabricated, they join the chase to keep pace with their own and others' intrigues. They press on out of fear that the number of followers and "likes" really does reflect social importance—a universal drive of tweens and teens.

Pertinent facts on teens and the Web:

• Cyberspace is part of the air that teens breathe. According to a 2015 Pew Research Center report, 92 percent of teens go online daily, including 24 percent who say they go online "almost constantly."[5]

• Almost 75 percent of teens have smartphones, which drives most of their Internet use. Of these, 58 percent say that they prefer to text when communicating with their closest friend.[6]

• According to a 2016 study by Common Sense Media, 50 percent of teenagers describe themselves as addicted to their mobile devices, while 27 percent of parents admit to feeling the same way.

• Teens are all about social interaction and the Web is yesterday's mall. Girls love to share creations, tell stories, and express themselves. They continue to dominate the blogosphere, but boys are more likely than girls to make friends online: 61 percent of boys, compared to 52 percent of girls, said they made friends on the Internet and they mainly do so through gaming.[7]

• Researchers continue to assess the impact of media exposure on teams. Prominent studies have shown no direct harm to either teens' social development[8] or brain development.[9] Nonetheless, recent research has suggested that heavy use of social media may be associated with teen suicidal behavior.[10]

Family Story: Caught in the Web of a Cyberstalker

At basketball camp the previous summer, 14-year-old Gabriella formed a friendship with a 20-year-old male coach. Since Gabriella's parents monitor her cell phone through spot checks, Gabriella and her coach agree to communicate during the fall through a private Gmail account and pre-arranged phone call dates. Flattered to have an older boy interested in her, Gabriella basks in his support and advice, particularly since she is starting a new school with few established friends. But after a while, he begins talking in more sexual terms about how attractive and hot she was last summer and how turned on he'd been by her athletic body. His emails become increasingly more graphic as he shares his erotic fantasies about her. He broaches the subject of meeting up, begging her not to tell her parents, because it would get them into trouble.

Confused, Gabriella begins backing off. When she tries to cut off emailing, he presses her harder, telling her how much he likes her and how sad it makes him that she won't get together with him. As much as she enjoyed his friendship and felt special because of it, Gabriella is distressed and frightened by the way he is pursuing her.

Having kept this dilemma secret, Gabriella finally breaks down and confides to a friend, who, in turn, shares the situation with her mom, who wastes no time before phoning Gabriella's mom.

Learning of Gabriella's situation, the mom is panicked and ready to see this young man put behind bars. The high pitch of her voice reveals her upset.

"Why did you keep this to yourself?" she cries. "I've told you that you can share anything with me if you're in trouble. I could have helped you. All you had to do is not reply to his emails!"

Mom moves into action, explaining that this is criminal behavior. "You're 14, and he's 20. We need to report this immediately to Child Protective Services, because he has no business working as a coach."

She's right, of course. Because of the age difference and because he persisted despite Gabriella's request to stop, it will need to be reported. But where does Mom's agitated response leave Gabriella?

A Calm Approach: Gabriella's situation illustrates how impossible it is for parents to cover every potential harmful situation. How many of us would send our kids off to a place as wholesome as basketball camp and say, "By the way, don't give your email address to your cute coach who you think is the coolest guy ever"?

Like cyberbullying, cyberstalking is covert and usually under the radar screen of parents. Before the Net, stalkers phoned their prey and showed up at school or a teen hangout, and adults were more likely to become aware of it.

Although he sounds sincere about caring for Gabriella, the coach's actions still qualify as stalking. If she had met him and they'd had sex, it would be statutory rape. Parents fear the anonymous stranger entrapping their child, but stalkers are more likely to be someone the teen had contact with (a friend of a friend) through parties or hanging out somewhere. For anyone in this dilemma, it's difficult to identify when all the flattery and attention crosses the line. Gabriella's situation is classic: The coach complimented her, supported her like a best friend, then slowly shifted ground, introducing sexual innuendo, wooing her with promises of love, and reeling her into a very scary place. Girls who are very needy for love and romance are more susceptible to this kind of setup.

It's critical for Gabriella to understand that none of this is her fault and that it could happen to anybody. Gabriella feels responsible, but the coach took advantage of a vulnerable, needy, and naïve girl, failing to respect her limits and then guilt-tripping her when she tried to pull away. This is a classic setup for some sweet, sincere girls who are trained to be polite, leaving them unprepared to defend against sexual advances.

For teens in a jam, parents can encourage them to trust their gut: "When you started feeling uncomfortable, that was a good sign that something unacceptable was going on." Also remind teens to be suspicious when someone swears them to secrecy and says not to tell their parents.

Gabriella's parents should let go of the mistake she made in keeping this to herself and commend her for what she did: "You were brave to tell your friend, and she had the courage to tell her mom. I hope this shows you we can handle this kind of situation without freaking out."

Parents can be perplexed when their teens clam up about a difficulty. But who wants to spill information that might get them into trouble or send parents into a tailspin? While some teens are surprisingly open, we shouldn't be at all surprised if teens share their embarrassments, vulnerabilities, and crises only with great reluctance. Keeping information from parents is normal, and we did the same!

Pertinent facts on Web safety:

• Despite publicity about online predators who prey on children by lying about their age and intent, the most common scenario involves a known older person who moves the conversation to promises of romance and love. Nonetheless, one in five U.S. teenagers using the Internet reports that they have received an unwanted sexual solicitation, asking them to engage in sexual activities or talk, or to give out personal sexual information. Only 25 percent told a parent. In 100 percent of the cases, teens who are the victims of sexual predators have gone willingly to meet with them.[11]

• Like social cruelty and peer victimization in the real world, these vicious actions are now played out in the same way in the shadows of the Web and can be more diabolical because they can be anonymous.[12]

• Although kids have always been reluctant to share uncomfortable social information with parents for fear of getting in trouble or setting in motion consequences that are disagreeable to them, there is a unique component with reporting cyber stalkers or peer bullying. They fear that parents will ban them from the Internet, which may be their tether to their social world.[13]

• Demographic and behavioral characteristics of teenagers are stronger predictors of online abuse than simply having an online profile. Girls and those who post large amounts of personal information online are more prone to online harassment.[14]

Family Story: **The Plague of Plagiarism**

A sophomore in high school, Aden is a conscientious, high-achieving student, respected by his teachers, and taking all honors classes. The family shares a desk area, and when Dad sees an English paper with an A on it, he decides to read it. Even though English is Aden's top subject, this paper is impressive. Then something catches Dad's eye. By chance, Aden has left his laptop open, and Dad finds evidence of an email exchange for the purchase of a paper from a clandestine website in Indonesia that wouldn't be detectable by normal school systems.

Dad is horrified and heartsick. Had Aden's plagiarism been discovered by the teacher, his A in the class would be ruined for sure, putting a big black eye on his report card and destroying his stellar GPA.

When kids are in serious trouble, parents will naturally feel protective and want to keep it contained. We all want our kids to have strong character, but not too many parents are willing to do the hard thing that exposes their teen and lets the difficult natural consequences unfold.

In this situation, Aden's dad is no exception, and he is tempted to spare his son and the family the embarrassment of going public. Dad's impulse is to deal with Aden directly, scaring him and setting him straight with a strong reprimand.

The problem is, Aden seems to have done this before. For a paper a couple of years ago, Dad caught Aden copying phrases from books, but he explained it away, claiming that it was just a rough draft. Dad wonders, will a serious scolding nip it in the bud? Is there a more important character lesson about cheating to be learned here?

A Calm Approach: Academic honesty is falling by the wayside as students experience more pressure to perform, and the Internet makes it easier to lift content. Parents need to be aware of how much cheating goes on and take it seriously. As with the subject of sex, not enough parents are talking to their teens about it. Teens are often impulsive, unaware of consequences, and prone to thinking that if "everyone does it," it's OK to cheat and fudge here and there, particularly when others leapfrog ahead dishonestly in class ranking.

Once Aden's dad comes to his senses, he realizes Aden hasn't mended his ways after the previous incident's strong lecture. His son needs to experience a bigger crisis. Sophomore year is as good a time as any for Aden to learn a lesson so hard that it will never happen again. Dad is disheartened to know that exposure will blemish Aden's record, and he has to face his own personal flaw for being tempted to value achievement over honesty for his son.

Confronting Aden, Dad makes him write an email to the teacher confessing his purchase of the paper. Aden receives an F and a good tongue-lashing from the teacher.

If not outright plagiarizing, parents are often guilty of overediting their children's papers, lending too much of a hand, often at the eleventh hour. Anxious for their kids to get good grades, parents don't see this as "cheating," and teens head off to college, still sending their papers back for parents to correct. Teachers can't teach their students if the work is that of their parents or the "ghost" on the Internet.

Pertinent facts on cheating:

• In a 2011 survey of 40,000 U.S. high school students, over half of the teens admitted to cheating on a test within the last year. One in three students owned up to plagiarizing an assignment using the Internet. The trend of academic cheating does not let up during college and may be connected to dishonesty later in life.[15]

• Good students, not just slackers, cheat, too. According to *Who's Who Among American High School Students*, four out of five high achievers who were surveyed admitted that they've cheated. More than half claimed that cheating was "no big deal," and almost none of them were caught.[16]

• The ease of downloading, searching, cutting, and pasting has blurred notions of authorship and loosened attitudes about borrowing others' words. Increasingly, as students work collaboratively in teams, notions of original copy and attribution fade. This practice may have contributed to a general slippage in ownership of material.

• Whether from rationalization or denial, many students lift material without including a citation, and this practice doesn't necessarily register with them as cheating. However, in college samples, when students are reminded of the importance of academic integrity and the nature of an assignment, cheating can be reduced.[17]

Family Story: **Pornography Invasion**

A funny thing happened to a mom on the way to her email. Waiting for her inbox to load, checking news headlines, she is startled when up pops a Web site with the most vivid, graphic, unattractive depiction of sexual relations that she has ever seen.

Mom is aghast. The only other person who uses her computer is her 12-year-old son, Hunter. Checking his browsing history, Mom discovers that the sweet little boy she is still sometimes tucking into bed at night has been surfing the Net, viewing pornographic sites, with whips, animals, multiple partners, and positions beyond her imagination.

It had occurred to Mom that "one day" during puberty she might have to address this topic. Instead, pornography has invaded her computer and their lives earlier than she ever expected.

Mom rushes to her husband and insists that he talk to Hunter about the twisted stuff he's viewing. Dad refuses. "Getting aroused with this kind of material is what healthy, red-blooded boys do," he says. "I did it with magazines; he's using the Internet."

"But this is really sick stuff," Mom insists. "There's a vast difference between *Playboy* a generation ago and what's readily available online today. What kind of impression do you think he's getting about sexuality from these sites? And these bodies—the breasts and the sizes of the organs are unreal. Don't tell me you think this is OK!"

"It's just sexual fantasy," Dad retorts.

"But he doesn't know that! It's so disrespectful of women. You've got to talk to him!" Mom screams.

A Calm Approach: Families typically divvy up sex-ed responsibilities by gender, with moms talking to daughters and dads to sons. But why not set gender aside and have moms and dads each express their views, allowing teens to get more than one perspective?

Hunter's parents have strong and different attitudes about pornography on the Web. Reacting to one another, they've ended up polarized. Each parent can have a talk with Hunter, but establishing ground rules and approaching it even-handedly are important. Dad isn't allowed to criticize Mom's position and vice versa. As an opener, each says, "I'm going to give you my thoughts, and I think it's important to listen also to [Mom's or Dad's] view."

Dad will be more understanding and less likely to shame his son for the interest in porn that he remembers so well. Nonetheless, when he speaks with Hunter, he's probably going to be a lot less approving of Net porn because he won't be in the midst of reacting to Mom's stance.

Both parents need to affirm their son's natural curiosity about sex and send a positive message on the role of sexuality in future healthy intimate relationships and marriage. But Hunter is being introduced to twisted and perverted versions of sexuality. Mom can stress that while Hunter's interest is normal, the images he's viewing are distortions. She can critique the objectification of women, the abnormal bodies, and depictions that have nothing to do with sexuality in a loving relationship.

All in all, they need to make sure Hunter is educated with other types of material, according to their values. They may decide to update their computer safeguards to make sure he is off pornographic sites.

Parents are rightly up in arms about porn on the Web, but take a look at ads and articles in mainstream media, particularly teen magazines. Sex is everywhere, used to sell even the most common products.

Common sense tells us what studies are showing: An American Psychological Association task force looked at a variety of media (TV, music videos and lyrics, magazines, movies, video games, the Internet) with respect to the "sexualization" of girls, that is, defining a girl's value exclusively on the basis of sexual appeal and behavior. The task force found links between this media and a plethora of ills in teenage girls, from eating disorders to low self-esteem to depression.[18] Equally alarming, the report finds that the trend toward sexualizing girls is on the increase as "new media" proliferates.

Teens are receiving lots of unrealistic, inaccurate, and misleading information about sex from the media. Be prepared for years of ongoing dialogue about media and sexuality, including your own attitudes and values in this area.

Pertinent facts on Internet pornography:

• Experts recommend that upon discovering a teen's use of porn, parents accept it as normal sexual interest and curiosity, while also voicing key concerns such as the following to their adolescent: Although sex education is vital, porn is a poor teacher, as it is usually presented without relationship context, storyline, or cues on sexual acts that ordinary people could replicate. Easy digital access can lead to compulsive viewing and a distortion of healthy sexual gratification. Real-life experiences may not measure up and brain chemistry associated with gratification may become altered. The industry often exploits both actors and viewers for "entertainment" profit, which can hurt the lives of all involved.

• A review of 135 studies examined the impact of exposure to pornography on women's and men's impressions of women as well as women's views of themselves. Evidence associates porn exposure with higher levels of women's body dissatisfaction; greater self-objectification (e.g. women's worth limited to sexual value); sexist beliefs; diminished views of women's competence and humanity; and greater tolerance of sexual violence toward women.[19]

• A review of the research on adolescent use of pornography has linked viewing pornography with girls feeling inferior and boys fearing their lack of virility. Teens seem to use porn less as they increase their self-confidence and sociability in the real world. Additionally, porn use is correlated with higher levels of conduct problems, depressive symptoms, and decreased bonding with parents.[20]

• Although Internet filters in the home do not shield tweens and teens from viewing pornography or disturbing online experiences, they are still recommended. They reduce the total amount of exposure, time usurpation, and "dosage" effect and send a strong message about parental values.[21]

Family Story: One-Click Shopping Goes Awry

Sixteen-year-old Brittany worships fashion. A label fanatic, she looks down on teens who don't wear the right brands and the trendy styles. To a great degree, her parents have gone along with her craze, buying her magazines, driving her to the mall, praising her good taste, while also overlooking her appetite for online shopping.

Most recently, Brittany has become fixated on purchasing a special handbag with her birthday money. On the hunt for just the right one, she settles on an expensive designer bag she locates on a website that looks legitimate. With a quick click but without consulting her parents, the purchase is made.

"Tragedy" strikes when the handbag arrives, and it is a cheaply made fake. Determining that this could be a tough but important lesson learned, Brittany's parents try to make her feel better about being deceived. "It's the least damaging thing that could have happened with this scam," they explain. "No one stole your debit card number or your identity." Inconsolable and insulted by their reasoning, Brittany pitches a massive fit.

Concerned at her loss of perspective, her parents wonder, "What have we wrought?"

A Calm Approach: Brittany's parents saw this incident as a wake-up call for circumstances that they had enabled. Too much of her time was going into image and exploring the Internet for fashion tips and purchases. We all like to look good, especially teens in the midst of fluctuating self-concepts, but Brittany valued almost nothing else, and her self-worth was based largely on the external.

Like many teens, Brittany had fallen deep into the trap of believing that she was better than others because she wore touted labels and trendy accessories. Insecure in their identities and desperate to fit in, teens—who represent billions of dollars of purchasing power—are hammered by marketing messages promising beauty and popularity. Values become distorted as esteem derives from owning certain things instead of substantive achievements, talents, and real-world relationships.

A courageous move, this family decided it was time for a new program that limited Brittany's exposure to shopping both on and off line, while also enhancing other talents. To be sure, Brittany would resist it and make her parents' lives miserable, but they resolved to stick together and stick it out. They would cease buying her things to please her. And most importantly, no longer would they turn a blind eye to the fact that she was purchasing items online, often using her parents' account without explicit permission.

As a family, they worked to become more media literate, including discussions on how to recognize online fraud. Brittany's parents shared their ambivalence about the blessings and curses of online shopping, delivering a needed item to the doorsteps overnight, while also making this all too easy.

All parents should emphasize the importance of being "marketing smart," discussing and modeling a resistance to the powerful forces that sway us to hand over our credit cards. If put to the task, teens can be adept at critiquing how commercials prey on insecurities and manipulate people into buying, but their budding identities render them vulnerable. Run a search on "how to market to teens," and you'll find Machiavellian techniques for persuading teens that they can be cool, likeable, and have more social power by buying stuff. It's not only online that teens are susceptible; the same pressure to purchase can happen at the department store make-up counter.

Our culture is notorious for buying into "more is better." As soon as we become used to one level of consumption, we strive for the next, never quite satisfied that enough is enough. We rail at how our kids want more, more, more, but as adults, we need to lead the way by putting a check on this all-too-human impulse.

Pertinent facts on teen consumerism:

• While broadcasting media has restrictions for advertising to kids, the Internet is unregulated. Sophisticated software collects data on teens' and our online searches and purchases and then targets advertising. Cyberspace is this era's mall where kids go to hang out, socialize and see what's cool. Marketers take full advantage.[22]

• The Web is rife with scams, fake ads, and fraudulent retail sites resembling the real thing. "Deals" arrive in inboxes by the dozens. Remind teens, if it looks too good to be true, it probably isn't.

• After research documented the significant buying power of teens, marketers began to target teens relentlessly. Marketers know that once teens identify themselves with a product and feel enhanced by this identification, it increases their spending. The message sent to teens is that by purchasing certain products they will acquire importance and group esteem, and all their problems will be solved.[23]

• Dubbed "pester power," marketers try to get kids to nag their parents to buy them stuff. Studies show a correlation between advertising and family conflict; the average young person said they have to ask nine times before their parents let them have what they want. This nagging pays off: Fifty-five percent of kids surveyed said they are usually successful in getting their parents to give in.[24]

• The trend toward greater materialism in teens does not bode well for their mental health. Values placed on service and strong connections with others result in greater purpose and life satisfaction, while a singular focus on financial aspiration is correlated with depression and anxiety.[25]

Family Story: Game Washed and Brain-Drained for School

Obsessed with brutal online war games, 14-year-old Ryan devotes hours on end to gaming with friends in his room as well as competitors across the globe. Early on, his parents had encouraged him to develop his computer skills. A little quirky and a bit of a loner, Ryan was previously without friends, despite his parents' efforts to engineer opportunities. But now, he hangs out with a group of fellow players who proudly call themselves "geeks." Concerns about the violent nature of the games notwithstanding, Ryan's parents see more upside than downside to this interest.

Although his parents are delighted that he at last has buddies, Ryan is becoming increasingly isolated from the family, spending more and more time in his room. When his parents question his hours spent online all evening, Ryan explains that he is nearly always doing his homework and just taking an occasional break to check for updates and reviews on new games. Since most schoolwork is now done online and is paperless, Ryan's parents go along with what he says, assuming that the greater share of his significant screen time is devoted to completing his assignments. Because he has been a decent student up to now, his parents have no basis for distrusting him.

Mid-term comments arrive, revealing that Ryan is failing multiple courses and has been lying about doing homework. Ryan's parents are stunned. They wonder whether they should prohibit all gaming because of its negative impact on school, but if they do so, he will lose his only friends, since online competition is their sole shared activity. They also have to admit that his self-esteem has improved because of his success and steady climb in the rankings.

"Gaming is everything to him. If we take it away, he'll revert to a friendless position and become depressed," they worry, "but this addiction is causing him to fail, and he has been lying to us!"

A Calm Approach: Many families share this predicament: Teens complain about having hours of homework and disappear behind closed doors. Instead of focusing on their work, teens stay connected to multiple sites and devises, splitting their attention and distracting them from the task at hand. Schoolwork suffers, and they get insufficient sleep. The approach for Ryan's parents and others is to tackle this problem as a team.

Although getting a teen like Ryan back on track will have many ups and down, most teens don't want to fail. They realize at some level that it's in their best interest to forge an agreement with their parents. Ryan would now do all his homework in the living room with his parents, turning over his cell to his parents so he wouldn't be distracted. With young children who have academic or impulsivity problems, parents can sit nearby to make sure homework is done, but guard rails of this restrictive nature are only appropriate for teens when absolutely necessary and with their buy-in.

Since Ryan was a whiz with computers, his parents realized the importance of a partnership with him instead of trying to manage his Internet use. The problem with media tracking and blocking systems is that teens can easily undermine parental controls by finding back doors and work-arounds. Smart high schoolers may even enjoy the challenge as a new form of a computer game!

Ryan's parents also enforced a strict bedtime limit and removed all devices from his bedroom at that time. Electronic devices emit light of a blue wavelength, which works against the release of melatonin, the natural sleep hormone. Tweens and teens with problematic screen habits stay up later, keep their cells on, awaken and respond to texts and snaps, and develop significant sleep-debts. Because sleep is so important to good health, savvy parents resist the classic teen spin of "having to stay up longer to finish homework!" The homework may very well be incomplete at the set bedtime, but it is virtually always the result of online touring in the bedroom, not the fib that they actually did six straight hours of homework.

Although Ryan's parents were horrified that he deceived them about doing homework, kids will lie—sometimes a lot—to keep their parents off their back. School work is a burden, compared to the dopamine-rich digital world of social networking and entertainment, offering escape and a means of coping with stress. The draw is just too compelling to expect teens to be entirely honest about their media use. Trust is a nice concept, but verifying is more realistic.

Monitoring school performance and screen time can be labor intensive, whether it involves checking an online system or emailing with teachers, but it's worth it if your child's school achievement is going downhill. If school performance is adequate but could be better according to your hopes, then you may or may not decide to "pick this battle." Kids understand interventions when school failure is on the line, but if battling over insisting on straight A's, you'll have less leverage.

To offset Ryan's obsession with gaming, he agreed to join one outside activity, in this case ultimate Frisbee. In return, his parents agreed to allow online competing, but at set times with certain parameters. His parents went online with him, and even though they objected to the blood and gore of some of the graphics, they marveled at his abilities and strategic skills. They agreed that they would pay for a summer computer camp, as long as he also went to a sports camp that restricted technology access.

His parents linked privileges on the weekend with responsible school performance during the week, and they allowed him input into which specific perks would be tied to what level of academic performance. For a strategy of this kind to work, parents need information about completion of assignments and test results every week. To be expected, there were a lot of setbacks in this process for Ryan and his family. Sometimes he would sneak around and devote more excess hours to gaming. He could be obstreperous and moody. Sometimes he blew off his homework and became angry when his parents took away his agreed-upon privileges. But with good work habits and homework completion as goals, Ryan's grades improved over time. Media is often rightly blamed for its power to distract but wrongly for its total responsibility for homework problems. Kids have been under-motivated and contemptuous of homework since the dawn of schooling, so "just turn it off!" flies in the face what we know about the tedium and the discipline needed to stay on task. Almost all kids—not just the ones like Ryan with technology-use problems — do homework with divided attention and wandering minds, yet despite the inefficiencies, they get it done, mostly.

Pertinent facts about Excessive Media Use Among Teens:

• As everyone can plainly see, cells and screens have dramatically changed the way that kids socialize, learn and play. As Jay Giedd, the adolescent brain scientist points out, this marks the biggest change in social interaction in five centuries, since Gutenberg's popularization of the printing press.[26]

• Experts are at a draw on whether conclusive evidence exists to prove the negative effects of video violence on children. Some have issued a plea for concern regarding violent video games,[27] while others have summarized the benefits to teens by playing video games, including cognitive, emotional, social, and motivational advantages.[28]

• Playing, hanging out and chatting while gaming creates greater closeness with friends. When polled, 79 percent of teen online gamers say that when they play online it makes them feel more connected to friends they already know. That amounts to 42 percent of all teens, ages 13 to 17.[29]

• Media use at night among teens is associated with going to sleep later, getting less sleep, and having sleep difficulties, which in turn relate to depressive symptoms.[30]

• While "Internet addiction" is a controversial topic among clinical diagnosticians, compulsive users can suffer problems similar to any substance use disorder. Similar to other addictions, excessive Internet use can carry negative consequences across social, emotional and academic domains. When access is unavailable, withdrawal effects can occur, including feelings of anger, tension, depression, and the compulsion to expand use and consumption.[31]

• Research continues to examine the upsides and downsides of screen-time, but teen well-being is not thought to be related to moderate media use.[32] After all, some teens are coding, some are supporting friends, and some are actually doing homework with friends! Important factors to analyze are the content of the use, the vulnerability of the user, and the context of the using.

Why Face Time Matters

An old saying goes, "If you see someone without a smile, give him one of yours." Good, bad, or ugly, emotions are contagious. Even complete strangers can exchange smiles on the fly and enjoy a fleeting moment of human connection.

Breaking important ground, psychologist Daniel Goleman pulled together a vast body of information to explain to the general public the scientific basis for the brain as a social organ.[33] Our brains possess their own kind of wireless network, with mirror neurons reflecting what we see, hear, and otherwise detect. When two people are face to face, emotions are exchanged through parallel neural circuits activated within each person's brain. It's as if "I 'catch' your emotions and you 'catch' mine."

In short, the brain takes in and responds to whatever is nearby. Whether it's "buy, buy, buy," porn on the Web, online gaming, or the general onslaught of media, the wired world is taking over our teens' brains. Parents would be smart to look twice at all their teens' world and ponder the question: What kind of media experiences and commercial culture do I want my teen exposed to during this vulnerable and high-opportunity time of brain growth and development?

Surrounded by tech gadgets galore, our teens are spending less time face to face with others. Across the generations, we've seen changes in communication preferences, from talking in person, to telephoning, to emailing, to texting. Teens may be "connecting" with others more rapidly and frequently, but it's increasingly abbreviated through media, where code lingo and emoticons substitute for expressing ideas and emotions in person. Technology ramps up communication feedback. Being online with multiple people is highly stimulating. Despite the drawbacks, when you're young, immature, and awkward, chatting online can be a lot more fun than sitting in a room talking to each other.

Most social-skills development occurs in the physical presence of other humans. One recent study tracked the impact of banning screen-based media for sixth graders attending an outdoor summer camp. With more time to interact, after just five days, the kids could read emotional and nonverbal facial expressions significantly better than those who maintained their media habits.[34] Face to face, we sense others' feelings, picking up cues from voice tone and cadence, facial expressions, and body language for how to respond. Neuroscientists use the term "empathetic resonance" to describe the way that brains process and affect one another. When others hurt, we hurt, too, making us inclined to take care of each other. If screen activities monopolize their time, teens can become emotionally thwarted, without the exposure that helps them learn empathy, caring, and the whole gamut of human emotions.

Present—not to mention future—relationships can suffer when teens fail to learn to take the time to sit and listen to another's perspective. Through experience, we learn how to validate others' feelings, hold back on interrupting, and sometimes not talk. Teens grown accustomed to high-speed stimulation can't tolerate the slightest whiff of boredom. When teens want to be wired to everything all the time, the simplest of activities—sitting quietly with your own thoughts—can become the rarest.

Now that American culture is saturated with mobile media, we find experts who think the sky is falling and others who think, the sky's the limit. Breakthroughs in technology put our values to test as we choose which opportunities to seize and which experiences to avoid. On the plus side, for example, we can stay in touch with our kids like never before. Over the Internet, shy kids who feel awkward in social settings can practice communicating in a way that creates less anxiety. Still, it's those face-to-face conversations that foster teens' social and emotional development and truly enrich our lives.

Parents grapple with myriad challenges created by our media-driven world. Diverse though the challenges may be, the common solution often comes down to parents overseeing the quality of their tween's or teen's screen use and enforcing some limits. Media use can stay in bounds if we reduce the opportunity for overdoing it. Ideally, once our kids finish their classes and after school activities, have dinner with family, do their homework, and go to bed at a reasonable hour, there's not enough time left over for heavy media use. Most teens can run circles around their parents with technology, but we still need to be supervisors, role models, mentors, and protectors as we all explore this rich and amazing realm.

CHAPTER 10

When Romantic Sparks Begin to Fly

The Teen Brain in Love

A couple of young teenagers begin noticing one another in a special way. They exchange texts — perhaps a friendly "What's up?" or a silly photo. Sometimes, a friend plays ambassador, "Jon likes you and wants to know if you want to hang out." From the initial bid to the closing of the deal, most parents are the last to know of their tween or teen's romance. And when they do, the first thought that often leaps into a parent's mind is "They're starting to date. We should have the sex talk."

Worried about things progressing too far too fast, some parents move straight to the big sit-down, not realizing that sex and romance are related but separate issues. Parents need a calmer, less reactive approach to early love. Teens muse, yearn, wonder, and fantasize about pure romance much more than parents ever realize. Only too easily do we overlook all of these intense feelings and miss out on an opportunity to have a discussion about relationships, not just sex.

Every aspect of their new attraction raises new questions for teens. Wandering into the maze of romance a teen thinks, "I should text him" one minute, but rethinks the decision the next: "I should wait for him to text me." Phone calls can feel too intimate to teens, so they're not usually part of the early stage of pairing up anymore. And of course, every friend and teen blog has an opinion on playing hard to get. Although teens need and deserve privacy, we want to demonstrate an appreciation for their vulnerability and confusion. An empathic remark like "Love is wonderfully complicated, and nobody has all the answers" shows that we understand how a new, potentially overwhelming part of life has opened up to them.

Parents can make a lot of flub-ups when their teens start pairing up. Here are some of the big ones:

- Being asleep at the wheel, unaware that something special is happening in the teen's life, expecting all the same grades, same interests, and same use of time.
- Minimizing and making light of the relationship, writing it off as only "puppy love."
- Being intrusive, believing that you as a parent have a God-given right to know everything about the relationship.

- Jumping to the conclusion that it's all about sex.
- Failing to realize when a relationship has become increasingly more intimate and it's time to move from talking about relationships to talking about sex.
- Having a button pushed from somewhere (your past, present circumstances, your fears) and becoming dogmatic and controlling, throwing up roadblocks at every juncture, potentially driving the teens into a "Romeo and Juliet" situation.
- Getting a vicarious thrill from your teen's romance and treating the boyfriend or girlfriend as if they're part of the family, inviting them into the home and including them in everything.

Falling in love is an experience like no other. A brain in love resembles a brain on cocaine. Using neuro-imagery, researchers have compared two groups: young people in love looking at photos of their loved ones, and young people who are not in love looking at photos of friends. Scans of their brains show distinctly different neural activity. When those in love gazed at their loved ones, the thinking part of the brain (prefrontal cortex) was less active, but the midbrain reward system, where addictive drugs and romantic love exert their powers, was activated. The pattern was not that of sexual arousal, but more like a dopamine flood.[1]

From a neurological point of view—and most of us would attest to this—falling in love is a big high, because dopamine (a neurochemical in our brains responsible for pleasure) is surging. The reward center in the emotional brain is hitting the euphoria jackpot, creating a desire to get high again! Be with this loved one as much as possible!

Most of us also know, or perhaps remember, the sensation of being so enthralled as to feel actually "lovesick." A biological basis for this pining and yearning exists. As noted, dopamine is increased, providing the sensation of profound pleasure. But serotonin (the brain chemical responsible for well-being) is decreased, which can lead to more sadness, more obsessing, and less contentment. At the same time, norepinephrine (adrenaline) is elevated, causing the heart to race, the appetite to fall off, and sweat to drip like a leaky faucet. No wonder anyone can be a mess when falling in love! This impact is even more magnified with naïve adolescents.

Sustaining the intensity and thrill of early love is impossible, for teens or adults alike. Young teens' relationships typically last only a few weeks or months, though by age 16 they can have more staying power. Still, discounting love between young teens as a "silly crush" is unfair and inaccurate, given the strength of teens' emotions. Rather, we need to take it seriously, understand the biological bases of their behavior, and appreciate the powerful mechanisms involved in pair bonding, which are hard-wired into our species and vital to its survival.

While the negative consequences from both broken hearts and sexual activity are legion, researchers also document the upside. Love not only makes you feel good, it can also be a buffer against pain, stress, and the blues. Many argue that positive social and emotional adjustment in adulthood stands on the foundation of what went well or didn't go well in romantic relationships during adolescence.[2]

Aside from the inevitable wrong turns, detours, and dead-ends in our teens' romantic journeys, what might, in the end, have a bearing on the relationships our kids are likely to forge? Parents can have a positive impact on what happens by maintaining a healthy relationship with their teen. Research shows that the quality of the attachment between parent and child influences the quality of teens' dating relationships, which, in turn, influences teens' capacity for long-term, committed relationships.[3] Forecasting about love is a dicey business, but teens who feel supported and secure in their relationships with their parents, gaining insight from them into the ways of the heart, can potentially build their future relationships on this secure foundation.

Family Story: **A Mom Fears Her Son Is Falling for a 'Fast Girl'**

On average, girls mature biologically about two years earlier than boys. Particularly in eighth and ninth grades, the physical differences can look spectacular! This gap means that girls, ever more sophisticated than boys, can come across as looking, sounding, and acting "fast," as they flirt, cajole, and mastermind their own and others' romantic pairings. Boys in their early teens often enjoy some of the attention and status, but can be confused about what girls want and what is expected in the pairing-up process.

Wary of the "little sluts," some moms feel very protective of their naïve sons. Debra was one such mom. Throughout her son Barry's years in middle school, Debra was relieved that he had steered clear of romantic entanglements, going with his buddies to the dances, and confiding in his mom that he didn't want the pressures of being someone's boyfriend.

Upon entering ninth grade, the tables have suddenly turned, as Barry becomes more guarded about his romantic life. What Debra suspects becomes apparent when she picks Barry up from his first high school dance and sees his classmate Alicia hanging all over him. Casually, she asks Barry what is up with Alicia. He replies with the line teens use to try to throw their parents off their romantic trail, "We're just friends."

Inquiring about Alicia to a friend, Mom discovers Alicia's questionable reputation. Moreover, Alicia has just been dumped by her older boyfriend, Matt, and has her sights set on Barry as her new conquest. Parents can seek helpful information from other parents, but figuring out what to do with the information is another matter. Good-looking and sprouting his first beard, Barry is a sweetheart, but Mom knows that he has the sophistication of a child when it comes to "hotties" like Alicia.

After the dance, the relationship appears to shift into a higher gear. Barry is breaking family rules about phone use late at night; there are many text messages to Alicia's number on his cell phone record; and he is becoming harder and harder to pin down about who is included in his group activities. The cagier Barry becomes, the more concerned Debra becomes about Alicia's influence. Keyed up, Mom wants the lowdown, but Barry is withholding, and it all comes out wrong in this conversation.

Content *(what is said)*	Process *(underlying dynamics)*
Barry: Mom, I'm riding my bike down to the store to check out some new headphones.	*Debra might have been more bugged by Barry's "announcing" instead of asking permission, but she has a bigger question on her mind about a secret rendezvous.*
Mom (Debra): Who are you going with or meeting up with?	*Although Debra is merely asking one of the basic questions about whereabouts, now that Alicia has entered the picture, she can't hide the question's heavy ring.*
Barry: Nobody. Why are you always asking me that?	*As legitimate as this parental inquiry is, Barry has detected a different tone, which annoys him.*
Mom: My "mom radar" tells me that you might be meeting up with Alicia. I know you told me that you are not dating her, but the grapevine suggests that you are.	*This sounds innocent, but Mom is now in trouble and should hold off, not push ahead. By not accepting Barry's "nobody" as the truth, she is implying that he's lying.*

Content *(what is said)*	Process *(underlying dynamics)*
	She has good reason to suspect it's "somebody," but pointing a finger puts him on the defensive.
Barry: Grapevine? Mom, really? Are you talking to the moms of all the girls again? Girls love to gab to their moms. Don't you moms have anything better to do than gossip about your kids?	*On the one hand, the mom grapevine can be an invaluable source of information. On the other, it can fan the flames of gossip as furiously as in a teen group. Debra would be smarter to safeguard this information for now because, from the tone of their exchange, Barry is not open.*
Mom: Look, Barry, I've tolerated just about enough of your acting like there is nothing going on, when you and Alicia texting constantly. And you know we have an agreement that I can look at your cell records. Will you please come clean with me?	*All parents have their breaking point for staying cool, calm, and collected, and Debra has reached hers. Having exercised patience for the sake of Barry's privacy and new love interest up to now, she has had it with his dismissals and evasions, and blows her cool.*
Barry: Mom, you are such a snoop lately, lurking by my door, always reminding me of my cell rules, and interrogating me about everything. It is really creepy. What's wrong with you?	*According to Barry, his mother has been transformed into a spy. In spite of Debra's view of herself as patient and respectful, Barry feels violated. There is validity to both views, but the chasm between the two leaves them disconnected.*
Mom: Barry, I am just looking out for you. Don't you know Alicia's reputation? She is sexually way out there. Has it ever occurred to you that she is just trying to make Matt jealous, and as soon as he's interested again, she'll drop you flat? I	*This is one of those times when even if you are completely right, you "lose" as a parent. Mom tries to defend herself by offering more evidence and emphasizing valid concerns, but she's digging herself a deeper hole by leaking her*

Content *(what is said)*	Process *(underlying dynamics)*
don't think you're ready for this!	*worst fears and badmouthing the girlfriend, which will fail to do anything except harm her relationship with Barry.*
Barry: Mom, you don't even know her! I can't believe you are talking such crap about her when you've never even met her!	*Debra has slipped into the trap of her own hypocrisy. Having taught her son to never spread gossip, she loses her personal credibility by maligning Alicia.*
Mom: I'd love to meet her, but you refuse to talk honestly about her, introduce me, or invite her over.	*Debra would be better off apologizing and trying to retreat by "owning" her overprotective zeal, but she's too upset to realize it.*
Barry: AS IF I would invite her now! Why would I introduce her to someone who hates her? That's the last thing I would ever do!	*Emotional buttons are pressed for mother and son, so Barry now perceives his mother's protective anxiety about Alicia as "hate." Considering what has been said, his reaction is understandable.*

Debra stops short of calling Alicia the names floating in her mind— "vixen," "slut," and "manipulative user"—but not by much. An anxious mom, she has imagined worst-case scenarios for Barry: Alicia will seduce her son and lead him down a wayward path of negative social influences. Then, she'll rip his heart in two, sending his grades and mental health into the tank.

Like a dam waiting to burst, Mom has pent-up news about Alicia. But unlike some kinds of information that always need to come out (threats of suicide or drug use, for example), what Debra knows isn't critical to her son's well-being. She wants a close relationship with Barry, but she won't get one by being intrusive. Her emotions running high, Debra blurts out her worries, which alienates Barry and could lead to more lying to and deceiving Mom and more closeness with Alicia. No matter how Debra tries to dig herself out of this mess, it's going to be a very long time before Barry trusts her with issues of his heart.

At this point, Debra's best option is to apologize profusely. She can express regrets that her protectiveness interfered with her faith in him to handle a romantic relationship as well as any intelligent ninth-grade guy with an attractive, confident young woman (leaving out "which is not very well!"). Debra needs to edit out put-downs of Alicia. Focusing instead on her connection with her son, she can discuss the need for compliance with family rules and honesty about his activities, but grant him leeway to navigate the tumultuous waters of romance without her interference.

Romantic relationships with the "wrong" partner can trigger anxiety in parents. Propelled by bad nerves, parents engage in behaviors that feel intrusive to teens, but parents defend as their responsibility. "Isn't it my job to protect my child if he could end up devastated and heartbroken?" a parent will ask.

In this kind of dilemma, questions to consider are: What is my goal? Is it realistic? How will I accomplish it? Even if a parent gets the benefit of an "I told you so," it's unrealistic to try to block every questionable romantic experience, and doing so undermines one of our ultimate parenting goals: to maintain connection, trust and influence, and enhance the likelihood that our teens will come to us if there's a problem.

Do's and Don'ts of Teen Dating for Parents

When teens' heart strings are tugging toward a new love, it can feel as if they're stretching away from parents. One common mistake is confusing teens' need for privacy with distancing. Teens in love will naturally become preoccupied with their romantic partner, needing space to explore the relationship. Still, we want to keep the parent-child bond healthy and intact, and here are some tips for doing just that.

Be respectful of your teen's relationship choices. As with teen friendships, reserve judgment unless you have hard-and-fast accumulating information that this relationship puts your child in harm's way. We can never be exactly sure what draws two people together or how long it will last. Bite your tongue and bide your time when you have reservations about your teen's new love interest, since mismatched alliances have a way of dying a natural death, given time.

Be careful about giving advice. Parents often feel teens need their counsel or are flattered by being asked for advice, but it's better to pose questions and let your teen weigh each option. Obsessing all evening with a teen over a romantic situation implies that you approve of a high level of preoccupation with teen love life. Do you?

Beware of trying to rescue your teen from hurt and heartbreak.
Although parents usually have more insight into a teen's love interest and the mess that can come from full-on heartbreak, warnings tend to come across as patronizing and condemning. Use "I" statements and focus on the positive. For example, instead of inflammatory responses like "He's bad news, I can tell!" try "I'm sorry if I've come across as untrusting or suspicious, but since he has refused to meet me, I haven't had a chance to get to know all the things you like about him."

Let the relationship be special and let it be theirs. A teen's first love could be the first time that parents feel really left out of their child's world. On a conscious or unconscious level, it can send the signal that the teen will, someday, form a bond with another loved one and fly the nest. Parents sometimes use their need to talk about sex as a back door into the teen's romance or to just plain get nosy. Our role pertains to concrete infractions that may arise out of the relationship, not the romance per se.

Encourage teens to be forthright about their relationships through win/win solutions. When teens are being cagey about their love interest, show a willingness to facilitate their needs in exchange for candor and compliance with family policies. Parents can say something like this: "Let's make a deal: You are honest, well-mannered, and respect the house rules, and I will do what I can to accommodate your desires to have time and space for a relationship that is important to you." This doesn't mean agreeing to all of their demands, but it encourages teens to be less secretive.

Appreciate the learning curve of romance. Don't forget that like any other skill area, teens need experience and practice in matters of the heart. Bumps and bruises allow teens to gain an understanding of themselves in relation to the people to whom they're attracted. Like any messy aspect of identity development or social and emotional competency building, parents need to accept that learning involves mistakes, hardships, and real experience.

Remember that this isn't a joking matter. It's astounding how parents can sometimes believe that young love is fair game for poking fun. "Oh, I notice you're taking more showers!" Or, "Wow, look at that new hair-do.

We know who you're seeing tonight!" Teens are going through one of the most vulnerable transitions imaginable, and we need to be sensitive, instead of yukking it up at their expense. If they look flushed after a phone call or are spending lots of time in the bathroom, better to act like we don't even notice.

Socializing, Romance, and Going Out

Establishing reasonable family rules early on about socializing, romance, and going out has clear advantages. By addressing inevitable policy issues up front—before a girlfriend or boyfriend is in the picture—you won't come across as "anti" the current love interest. If you spring restrictions on them when they're under the influence of love, they may accuse you of just not wanting them to date or not liking their mate.

Parents may disapprove of many things their teens push for: "I won't go on the vacation unless Tom can come!" "Why can't we be in my bedroom together? We're just listening to music." "I'm only going to have a few friends over while you're out." Sometimes parents concede to teens' questionable agendas because they want to be popular with their teens or they're hoping to enhance their kid's popularity. Other parents prefer a level of ignorance about their teen's romantic life, as if "what I don't know, I don't have to do deal with." But ignorance can be far from bliss, as parents sort out the challenges of family rules with teens who are wrapped up in romance.

Parents are often perplexed by the following issues:

Middle-school romances. By sixth grade, romance can be in the air, but teens still have seven years before they graduate from high school. There's an upside to holding back on middle-school dating, because it allows parents to extend more freedom over time, giving older teens the kind of leeway that is more appropriate for high school. Middle schoolers may begin "going out," an agreed-upon pairing up whose meaning ranges from practically nothing (half a day of hanging out together) to everything (long-term and maybe even intercourse). Although parents typically create policies according to their values and philosophies, most middle schoolers tolerate limits (no one-on-one dates, no regular chauffeuring to one another's homes, for example), so why start the clock on dating any earlier than necessary?

Boy/girl parties. Teens will push for these and may also try to set unreasonable parameters, such as "I don't want a birthday party unless girls/boys can come, and you can't come into the room, you don't need to know who is coming, and don't insist on meeting everyone." When parents are adamant about oversight, teens may accuse them of being a "control freak." Nonetheless, parents are responsible for supervising teens in their home. In the nicest way possible, let the teen know that you will be coming in the room now and then, and that you really would like to meet her friends. And if the party is in someone else's home, it's perfectly fine to phone the parents to make sure they're home, even if your teen pitches a fit.

Boy/girl sleepovers. Mixed-gender sleepovers among five best friends from elementary school are probably innocent, but the problem is determining the age at which this might cross over into something else. If you say "yes" in sixth grade, will teens expect it the next year? Special circumstances may come into play, but consider drawing the line early on this. If you phone other parents, you may find that they don't like this idea either and are dying to say "no," but don't want to be the first one to make the connecting phone call. Teens will push for coed sleepovers, particularly in high school after big events such as homecomings or the winter ball. A good option is for parents to organize an alternative, such as dividing teens into two sleepovers, one for girls and one for boys.

Public displays of affection. Different parents have different comfort levels about "PDA," but schools discourage, if not outright ban them, so parents should consider being consistent with school policies. Holding hands is one thing, but making out on the couch in front of others is entirely another. Parents can explain that this is about manners, decorum, and having a boundary between what's proper in a public versus private setting.

Dating an older teen. Generally speaking, healthy relationships among teens tend to occur between teens who are about the same age and not more than two years apart. Older teens are more likely to be sexually active and psychologically more mature, and will implicitly have more power over their younger partners.

Group socializing. Unlike the old days when teens "went steady," today's dynamics are different. Teens are more likely to travel in packs than in pairs. Parents can have a false sense of security from group activities, believing there's less likelihood of kids getting together as couples. Group activities can actually intensify romantic interest. Assuming safety in numbers, parents tend to ease up on supervising and tracking, leaving teens freer to pair up secretly and go off somewhere without parents having a clue.

We're "just friends." This may even be true, but hearts can flip-flop. Relationships often start off unclear and ill defined, with teens only knowing that they want to hang out and talk more. Then they kiss and realize it's something special, but they may not want to admit to a shift in the relationship because of the huge ramifications. If parents don't know the nature of the relationship, they don't know what their policies should be and how to supervise. Be advised that teens will often identify someone whom they have romantic feelings for as "just a friend," because parents let their guard down, allow more freedom, and ask for fewer details.

Something's afoot. What is it? Sometimes parents—almost always mothers—have a sense that something is going on. Teens are showing a lot of interest in one another, but it's not clear whether there's a romantic relationship and/or whether it's sexual. Could they be hooking up? Hooking up can entail anything from kissing to casual sex outside of a relationship. Because it does mean something sexual, most parents will want to weigh in with their values and health information. Parents who feel in the dark about their teen's love life can seek out information from other trustworthy parents.

When home alone gets complicated. Allowing teens of the opposite sex to be alone in the home together is a call parents can make based on how they feel about possible romantic trysts. The teens could be "just friends"—or they could be more. Many parents arrive home to discover teens in bed together and, in fact, most pregnancies occur in a teen's own home. Sometimes parents have gone about setting rules for when teens are home alone, but forget to reiterate them or just let them slide.

Open-door policies. Most teens feel as if they own their rooms and are entitled to have peers in with the door closed. If you're not comfortable allowing your teen to shut the door, make a preemptive move and set a policy before teens have a girlfriend or boyfriend. Teens will go on the offense and tell you you're obsessed with sex and that nothing is going on, but once the door is shut out of habit, it's harder to get it open again. If you've fallen for this ploy and the door is closed, go ahead and insist it be open, but be ready for a tussle.

Sexual identity. Many parents of teens who are gay have suspicions about their teen's sexual identity from an early age, but others either don't pick up on the cues or deny them. Even before relationships are part of the picture, pubescent teens can have inklings or a strong awareness of whom she or he is attracted to, and thus the "Who am I?" question enters the teen's mind.

If your teen does "come out" to you—disclose that he or she is gay—don't be too quick to declare that perhaps it's "just a phase." Maybe it is, but this reaction reveals a rejection of the possibility. As with any big news ("I want to drop out of school and join a band," "I don't believe in God anymore"), the best thing to do when your blood pressure skyrockets is "Don't just do something, stand there."

The same advice applies when teens come out as "bisexual," which can be a transition stage for uncertain teens, some of whom may realize they're gay later on. Or these days, it can be another way or exploring sexuality and sexual identity. Try to stay calm, get them talking, listen, and then study up on the subject so that you can stay connected to your child. Contact Parents and Friends of Lesbians and Gay Men (PFLAG), get a reading list, and consider going to a parent group. This will help immeasurably.

When we have babies, we almost always assume that they will be straight. Helping your tween or teen to become well-adjusted requires that we learn about parts of their identities that may be unexpected or may make them vulnerable in a world that marginalizes individuals considered in many sectors as "different," "other," or "less than." Even if your teen isn't gay, discuss this topic with your teens, because they will know someone who is, and you want to make sure that they treat that person with respect. Homosexuality isn't a disorder; national organizations of psychiatry and psychology removed it from the diagnostic manual decades ago. Some religious institutions deem it unacceptable, but the science of sexuality has determined that this is a naturally occurring variant of normal human sexuality, and it defines up to about 10 percent of people.

And what about the transgender identity — the "T" in LGBT? Transgender individuals have almost always felt themselves to be a different gender from that ascribed to them by their sexual parts, usually starting in toddlerhood. While the relative number of transgender tweens and teens is low, the harms they may suffer during adolescence are serious, including violence, harassment, bullying, and suicide. The American Academy of Pediatrics has issued a statement in support of protection of the transgender community, which can be a talking point with all of our kids.[4] Busting out of old categories, young people may identify as everything from queer to fluid to asexual.

Downsides of Romantic Relationships

Extreme dependency. By high school, some teens spend so much time with their romantic partner that parents feel they only see their teens coming and going. Exclusivity is a big downside of dating, particularly when teens want to drop all other socializing to be with their girlfriend or boyfriend.

One of the hardest patterns to witness is the teen, especially girls, who lower their expectations to get a boyfriend. In fact, research has documented that when girls deviate from their pre-conceived, idealized sequence of romantic progression—holding hands, exchanging "I love you's", etc.—they are more likely to become depressed.[5]

Understandably, many parents are unhappy when their teens put nearly all their eggs in the romance basket, instead of dividing their time and energy among sports, school, and a variety of extracurricular activities. Love is one of those phenomena that is not within a parent's power to direct or dictate. We can set limits on how many nights a week our teens can spend with their partner and try to keep them involved in other activities. Still, no matter how many rules we make around romance, parents can't control teens' emotions. No one plans to have their teen engulfed in a relationship, but it sometimes happens that way.

Dating abuse. Love evokes the best and the worst of our deepest passions and desires. Dating violence is defined as the physical, sexual, psychological, or emotional violence within a dating relationship, which also includes stalking. For adults and adolescents alike, romantic relationships can go seriously wrong, as research over the past decade has documented.

- Among adults surveyed, 22 percent of women and 15 percent of men who experienced rape, physical violence, or stalking by an intimate partner had experienced abuse by a partner before the age of 18.[6]
- Among high school students who dated, 21 percent of females and 10 percent of males experienced physical and/or sexual dating violence.[7]
- In a large-scale survey of high school students, 27 percent said they had had a partner who had called them names or put them down and 75 percent said that it is OK for a partner to be "really jealous" at times.[8]
- One in three girls between the ages of 16 and 18 say that sex is expected for people their age if they're in a relationship; half of teen girls who have experienced sexual pressure report they are afraid the relationship would break up if they did not give in.[9]
- Almost 20 percent of teenage girls who have been in a relationship said

a boyfriend had threatened violence or self-harm if presented with a break -up.[10]

Teens don't necessarily know what is right and wrong in dating relationships, and without some guidance, may tolerate dynamics that put them at risk. That's why it's so important for parents to maintain trust and connection in their relationship with their teen. Steering clear of unnecessary intrusiveness improves the odds that teens in a pinch will be open to parents' wise counsel.

For example, a boyfriend might constantly monitor his girlfriend's behavior, demanding to know what she is doing and with whom. This kind of jealousy could be interpreted by a naïve teen as caring, instead of one of the warning signs of abuse, something that should never be tolerated.

Schools and community-based organizations have recognized that dating violence is a significant problem that needs to be addressed in health educations classes to reduce dating abuse and deleterious patterns in emerging adulthood.[11] To stay safe and healthy in their relationships, teens benefit from information about gender stereotypes, conflict management, assertiveness skills, and non-violent communication. Advice for parents: Study up and look for opportunities to introduce these important topics in non-intrusive ways.[12]

Messy break-ups. Though split-ups occur all the time, they can be excruciating for teens. When break-ups get sticky, teens with trustworthy parents will often consult them—but usually not as early in the mess as the parents would like.

Teens can feel pulled in different directions when trying to end a relationship. They want it to be over, but feel terrible about shutting down the person they once cared for or even loved. Desperate to hang on, former partners can plead, "Just text or call me later. I just want to talk. Why won't you even talk to me anymore?"

Breaking up and getting back together can go on for months, as teens sort through guilt, confusion, and mixed feelings. Technology — texting and posting on social media sites — has made it all the more difficult to sever communication. Compassionate and reasonable parents see how miserable their teens are and may suggest the obvious solution—taking a break from accessing sites shared with the ex to tone down the break-up intensity and hard feelings. Most teens are too emotionally overwrought to cut these ties, as they often do want to track the activities of their ex. There are no easy solutions for "clean" break-ups in the digital generation. Real endings are messier than ever, especially since weak moments in the middle of the digital night can set the volume to high with the tap of a finger. Teens suffer when their former girlfriend or boyfriend tells them they're being mean and heartless. Reasonable parents can be wonderfully helpful to a teen struggling to call things off. Staying firm, compassionate, and empathetic, parents can reassure their teen: "People act in desperate ways when they feel rejected. It's so hard to be told you're cold, but stick to what you're doing because only time apart can lead to healing."

Parents can help their kids be realistic about what to expect: Teens who feel "dumped" can be angry and try to hurt back. And when your child is the one who is being dumped, he might need help with the tough work of grieving the loss and moving on. In either case, a note of caution for parents: Avoid overt badmouthing; the couple could be back together in a week.

The Benefits of Dating

Today's teens have plenty of reasons why they don't date. Just ask them and they'll tell you that dating involves too much drama, too much responsibility, and too much distraction from schoolwork. They don't want to get stuck with one person and lose their freedom. Most high schoolers would like to be in a relationship some day, but many have opted out for the same reason as college kids: They're too busy.

One-to-one dating has been on a downward trend over the past decades. Emphasizing school achievement, athletics, and other talents, many parents think that's great. Not dating means teens aren't communicating for hours every night with a boyfriend or girlfriend, stealing time from homework and résumé-building extracurricular activities. The problem is that even if dating relationships are on the decline, sexual attraction isn't, which is one reason why having sex outside of a relationship has become more common among teens.

Despite the downsides of romance—the potential for heartache and hurt or the drain on family, academic, and personal life—teens benefit more than parents might imagine from good old-fashioned dating.

What exactly are the upsides? On the simplest level, dating can be an opportunity for parents to reinforce manners: making a good impression, shaking hands with parents, looking grownups in the eye, accompanying a date to and from the door, being helpful in others' homes and respectful of whatever rules they have. Motivated to impress their date and the parents, teens may acquire good behaviors that once meant little to them.

Similar to challenges in sports (losing the championship), academics (doing poorly on a test), and friendships (having a significant disagreement), romance includes highs and lows. As parents, we want to help our kids have healthy, balanced relationships and to learn from whatever happens. Romance can make the strongest person feel vulnerable, as teens figure out how to manage emotions, rebound from disappointments, and recover from heartache.

Most parents hope that their teens will grow up to be successful in their careers and their love lives, but we don't give enough attention to what it takes to achieve happy, satisfying marriages. Romance can get in the way of grades, SAT prep, and family time, but it builds valuable skills. Being in a relationship helps teen become comfortable in the art of conversation; they learn about consideration for others' feelings, cooperation and mutual support, trust, empathy, sensitivity, and coping with all the emotions that stem from opening yourself up to another person.

Through romantic relationships, teens explore their identities and values, and discover what they like and dislike in partners: "I like a girlfriend who is ambitious and cares about school," "I like optimistic guys who aren't controlling and have their own lives," "I'm interested in someone who is fun, resilient, and kind to parents and friends."

Some teens will take another path in high school and not date at all. Parents don't need to worry or try to orchestrate dates; their teens are probably just on a different trajectory and can develop interpersonal skills through other activities. Temperament and personality impact how a social life unfolds, and a teen may simply not get around to dating until later in life. Being in love during high school doesn't go on a résumé and isn't as impressive as immersing yourself in ballet, the school newspaper, or volleyball, but it still shouldn't be overlooked as a worthwhile learning experience.

Teen romance is yet one more ingredient to drop into the stew pot of adolescent challenges. Unsure of what's bubbling up, parents have wildly varied reactions. Some parents feel anxious and protective, and interfere in inappropriate ways. Others view teen love as cute and try to expedite it. Lots of parents disapprove, believing that teen romance and dating leads to nothing but bad news and pulls teens away from activities that keep them on the straight and narrow. Some parents don't acknowledge their teen's love life at all, while still others experience so many uncomfortable feelings that they cope by poking fun. Parents need to be very thoughtful about their role and responsibilities in a teen's romantic relationships. As difficult as it may be, we have to give them privacy, refrain from interrogating them, keep a watchful eye without intruding, let them make mistakes, and be there for support during the tough times. Our responsibility lies in setting up reasonable policies and enforcing family rules.

When our teens fall in love, it can be another humbling moment of realizing that our kids are different from us. Their relationships are a window into who they are. Romance can be big and consuming for teens, and mystifying for parents. "What does she see in him?" a parent may ask. To this question, consider the astute words of 18th-century French philosopher Pascal: "The heart has its reasons, which reason knows not of." As true today as it was centuries ago, we can't always make sense of romantic choices, especially those of a teen in love.

CHAPTER 11

When You Need to Talk About Sex

Puberty Dawns

There it is, right before you: the waft of body odor, the crack in the voice, or the developing breast buds. Any number of telltale signs announce unmistakably that puberty is under way. Physical changes like these can unsettle teens and parents alike. Parents may feel some sadness, since teens' new bodies signal the beginning of the end of our childrearing years, though there's also much to appreciate and admire in their growing up. A son may start looking more like a man and be strong enough to mow the lawn faster than a parent. A daughter may begin developing muscles and curves, looking as beautiful in her volleyball team uniform as she does in a dress.

Timetables for puberty—when it starts and when it's finished—vary enormously among kids. The neuro-endocrine system stimulates the pituitary gland, sending a message to increase the production of sex hormones, specifically estrogen and progesterone in girls, and testosterone in boys. With increased levels of these hormones, puberty dawns.

As these powerful hormones interact with changes in the brain, mood swings in teens can be dramatic. Testosterone, which is barely detectable before age 10, can increase by 30-fold by the end of puberty. Despite assumptions, researchers have yet to find a direct link between testosterone in male teens and greater dominance, territoriality, and aggression.[1] The outbursts and reactivity that become more familiar to parents during the teen years do, however, appear to be related to testosterone release during puberty, according to recent research on teen brains.[2]

Estrogen is the primary female sex hormone, contributing to healthy bone growth, sexuality, and reproductive processes such as menses and fertility. Parents may become concerned if their daughters show signs of early puberty, sometimes as early as 8 or 9. Girls who mature early (developing breasts and pubic hair but not starting their periods) can be at increased risk for a range of psychosocial problems including depression, substance use, and early sexual behavior.[3] Nonetheless, the family can serve as an important buffer.[4] Parents can treat this bodily change in a positive, non-stigmatizing way, as they would with any other developmental change like getting taller or losing teeth.

With either gender, meltdowns can occur out of the blue. A parent may deliver laundry, but instead of receiving a word of thanks be met by a scream,

"Get out of my room!" A simple request to help unload groceries can trigger a show-down. Teens can sulk and weep or snap back impatiently at a parent's most innocent question.

One hundred and fifty years ago, menarche (the beginning of menstrual periods), psychological maturity, marriage, and childbearing all happened within a span of a couple of years, typically from ages 16 to 18. With everything under way around age 16, parents were spared the experience of living under the same roof with their teens and contending with an extended period of adolescent moods and mayhem. Children matured and then left home, assuming new relationships, roles, or occupations in one fell swoop.

Today, girls start having periods around age 12, which means that hormonal changes bringing about menstruation begin around age 10. Psychological maturity doesn't come about until the early to mid-twenties and most young people now postpone marriage until their mid- to late twenties.

A century ago, expecting young people to hold off on having sex until they were married may have been realistic, since it wasn't a very long wait. By contrast, most of today's adolescents have, roughly speaking, around 15 years from the time their hormones awaken sexual feelings and desires until they're married. Most parents realize that 15 years is a long time to repress powerful biological drives. This math makes the whole question of parental expectations for their teens' sexuality far more complicated. As young as it seems, on average, teen boys begin having sex at age 15 and girls at age 16.

New Bodies, New Challenges

On top of new emotions awakened by puberty, teens are also coping with exceedingly rapid body changes. With the exception of infancy, puberty is the human body's most accelerated period of physical growth. No wonder teens spend so much time before the mirror—they're changing right before their eyes! Only too easily can parents slip into jovial teasing about adolescents' new physiques, which is insensitive at best, if not cruel. Parents often aren't empathetic enough to how much teens suffer as they watch their noses grow and count their new zits. Analyzing their morphing bodies, teens wonder, "Am I normal?" "How do I compare?" "What do I look like to other people?" Obsessive mirror gazing is more about teen vulnerability than vanity.

Growth spurts can be dramatic; pants fit one day and stretch above the ankle the next. Or, a teen may be bothered by the opposite—being stuck in a little-kid body, not changing enough. Consider also the disproportionate maturation rate of girls versus boys. In general, boys lag about two years behind girls. Any given sixth-grade class contains a motley mix of girls with finely etched features and bodies growing shapely, towering over scrawny or pudgy boys.

A parent's job is to take the lead in supplying teens with copious information about what's happening to their bodies, whether it be menstruation, breast development, genital growth, or nocturnal emissions. Get books, sign up for classes together, and use every possible natural opportunity to reassure teens that what they're experiencing and feeling is a normal part of human development. Girls should know what's happening to boys and vice versa. Acne may be one subject about which teens will ask parents for help. Otherwise, most teens are too timid to approach parents about sensitive body issues.

Incredibly sensitive to their bodies, some teens start having body-image problems at puberty. Boys begin working out, worrying about muscles. It can be traumatic for boys if they're predisposed to very small stature, just as a larger body type can be devastating to girls. Less than 1 percent of the population has the body type of the average model, yet many girls believe they should look like the images on a fashion magazine cover, seeing beauty only in slender thighs, small waistlines, and tall statures. Wildly unrealistic in their expectations, they can feel demoralized by the increase in body fat and padding on the hips and thighs that appear right before they start their periods.

Body-image issues at puberty often lead to dieting, if not disordered eating. A survey of 80,000 high schoolers documented that more than 50 percent of girls and about 25 percent of boys engaged in some kind of disordered eating behavior, such as fasting, skipping meals, smoking cigarettes to curb appetite, using diet pills or speed, self-induced vomiting after eating, or using laxatives.[5] Restrictive dieting doesn't automatically lead to a full-blown eating disorder, but it can put teens at risk. And as usual, parents can make a difference. A large review found that family support and connectedness, regular family meals, and avoiding comments about weight gain are inversely correlated to teen eating problems.[6]

Nutrition is an area where parents can easily trip up. At one end of the spectrum are uninformed parents whose children need education on obesity; at the other end are controlling parents who think that with enough willpower, their kids can be thin. This harmful assumption sets teens up for disordered eating, because the body resists the effects of starving by instigating food cravings.

Genetically, people are predisposed to have a range of body weights. But our billion-dollar dieting and fashion industries have conspired to brainwash people into believing that through discipline and marketed products, a vulnerable teen can be thin and gorgeous and thereby cool, popular, and successful.

Daughters, in particular, may ask for help with diets, or parents may volunteer themselves to help. Under the guise of "helping" their teen "get healthy," parents can slip in comments that aren't helpful in the least, like "Are you sure you want that second helping of mashed potatoes? Aren't you watching your weight?" If parents believe that their teen needs to learn about carbohydrates, proteins, and fats, or portion control, they can say it once—only. Anything more can seem judgmental and critical.

As teens shed their little bodies during puberty and move toward more mature womanly or manly physiques, our job is to help them keep a healthy body image. Still, a parent's role in controlling a teen's food intake is limited. We provide healthy, well-balanced snacks and meals at regular intervals, but they choose what to eat and how much. Mandating some kind of physical activity for fitness is also a good move. Not just for staying fit and fending off obesity, exercise benefits teens all around, improving moods, self-esteem, confidence, and social competence. Otherwise, we keep our mouths closed, allowing our teens to be wherever they are on the body-type curve.

Talking to Teens About Sexuality: Myths and Misconceptions

Sexuality is one of those topics that most parents dread and avoid, to their teens' detriment. We know we should talk about it, but we feel embarrassed, awkward, and ill equipped. Most of our parents did a marginal job in this area, leaving us without role models for conversing about something as intimate and private as sexuality. And, secretly, we may prefer to hang onto an image of our kids as little innocents.

As with any highly charged area associated with big emotions, taboos, and discomfort, we cling to excuses that offer a free pass out of the dreaded task. Myths and misconceptions cloud our thinking.

Here are some of the big fallacies:

Telling my teen not to have sex is the most effective way to protect him or her from the negative consequences of sexual activity.

How nice to think that we could effectively advise our teens, "Just don't do it," but this doesn't work and never has. The brutal truth is that parents have influence, but not necessarily control over their teen's sexual behavior. As our children move increasingly outside of our orbit of direct supervision, we help keep them safe by maintaining a close relationship with them and enhancing their education and self-awareness.

I should hold off on talking to my teen about sex until there's a serious girl-friend or boyfriend in the picture.

Although parents should step up discussions about sexuality when teens are in relationships, the earlier the conversations occur, the better. Experts estimate that parents are two years behind where their teens need them to be with regard to sex education.[7] Only one out of three parents of sexually active 14-year-olds realizes that their child has had sex. By the time parents think, "I should talk to my teen," they've probably missed the opportunity to be most helpful.

A position paper from the Society for Adolescent Medicine recommends that teens should have the human right to information about their sexual health.[8] Most health experts agree that teens need sexuality education that teaches them refusal and negotiation skills, and gives them up-to-date information about birth control and sexually transmitted infections before they are sexually active.

I can rely on abstinence-only sex education at school to help keep my child safe and chaste.

Research has shown that abstinence-only sex education programs do not delay sexual initiation or reduce teen pregnancy.[9] By contrast, programs called "Comprehensive Sex Ed" include abstinence as part of the curriculum, but they also incorporate ways to prevent pregnancy and promote health. Whether at home or school, a comprehensive approach to sex education has been shown to result in better contraceptive practices for teens.

If I talk to my teen about sex, it will put the idea in his or her head, enhance curiosity, and increase the likelihood that sex will occur.

The data couldn't be clearer: Children whose parents talk with them about sex have no increased rates of sexual activity. And when they do become sexually active, they're more responsible about practicing safe sex. Research shows that teens with the most connected relationships with their parents have the most responsible sexual behaviors, including delaying intercourse, being less promiscuous, and practicing safe sex.

My teen squirms, rolls eyeballs, and practically runs for cover when I broach the topic of sex. This means that my teen really doesn't want to talk about this with me.

This kind of "go away" body language is another bizarre aspect of adolescence. In numerous surveys, teens say that they actually do want their parents to talk to them about sex. Parents will sometimes bring it up by asking, "Do you have any questions about sex?" Most teens will say, "No," and the parent replies with the lamest possible response: "Well, if you do, let me know." We should be the ones knocking on their doors. Teens may act reluctant, but parents need to make it their responsibility and take the initiative in this area—because teens probably won't!

Once I've had "the talk" with my teen, I don't need to continue bringing it up. After all, they get plenty of information from health-education classes at school.

Instead of having "the talk," parents should commit to an ongoing dialogue about sexuality from childhood to adulthood. Parents are in a unique position to customize their messages, targeting the right moment and teaching their values in a way that is relevant and approachable to their teen. What parents don't tell their teens about sex they will find out from peers and media—sources that may be distorted and misleading. Parents who prove themselves trustworthy and willing to wade into these choppy waters are more likely to have their teens come to them in times of need.

I don't want my daughter to have a boyfriend, because boys only want one thing: sex.

Stereotypes abound about sexuality, especially the one about girls yearning for love and boys craving sex. Testosterone in boys may, indeed, make them more driven sexually than girls, but it doesn't create a direct link. Likewise, girls' higher levels of oxytocin (sometimes referred to as the "tend and befriend" or "cuddle" hormone) motivate them to establish relationships. Nevertheless, many girls will push for sex, and many boys are forlorn and undone because they're head over heels in love.

Although girls and boys both have strong sexual impulses, boys are sometimes the ones to be more logical about contraception. In our culture, some girls are so conflicted about having sex that they feel more innocent if sex "just happens" in a moment of passion, as opposed to a premeditated decision. Guilt in girls doesn't prevent sex, but it can prevent proactive planning for responsible sexual activity and can be associated with unwanted pregnancy.

Because of our sex-obsessed culture, I assume that rates of sexual activity and pregnancy among teens have skyrocketed.

Sex is everywhere in our culture, but rates of teen sexual activity, pregnancy, and childbirth have actually dropped over the last decade. The prevalence of sexual activity is down significantly from 1998 to 2015, from 51 percent to 42 percent among female teens and from 60 percent to 44 percent in teen boys.[10] In 2010, the teen pregnancy rate reached its lowest point in more than 30 years, down 51 percent from its peak in 1990. Improved contraceptive practices have played a role in this trend. Recent research indicates that long acting, reversible contraception (LARC) methods like the IUD and the implant are proving to be extremely effective for preventing pregnancy.[11]

Approved by the American Academy of Pediatrics, LARC methods are considered the best protection against unwanted teen pregnancy because they require one procedure for protection for 5 to 12 years, instead of teens needing to plan ahead and take pills or use a method during intercourse (like the diaphragm or sponge) when in the swirl of emotions. Although LARC methods can prevent pregnancy, regular use of condoms to prevent sexually transmitted infections is also a must.

I believe that teens shouldn't be having sex, so it's a double message if I talk to them about safe sex practices and birth control.

These two separate messages can be put together without contradiction. In no uncertain terms, we can say, "I don't think teens should have sex, but if you do, you need to use a condom to prevent sexually transmitted infections along with one other form of birth control to prevent pregnancy." This statement doesn't condone sex, because the parent's position is very clear.

Consider the "but" clause as an insurance policy. We don't expect to have car wrecks or house fires, but if they happen, we have the policy in place. Or think of it as an immunization. We don't want our kids to have measles, so we prevent it through immunization. By talking to our teens about safe sex practices, we offer them "psychological immunization" against irresponsible sexual activity.

When talking to my teen about sexuality, I should focus mainly on the dangers, such as pregnancy, sexually transmitted infections, and sexual assault.

Parents should, of course, address various dangers associated with sexuality, which might bring them harm. But if we give only the "doom and gloom" spin on sex, what happens when teens find out that sex can bring incredible pleasure and the powerful emotional intensity of intimacy? When their experience doesn't match the dreaded threats of parental warnings, we risk our credibility. It's best to include the whole story on sex.

Family Story: Navigating the Tricky Waters of Talking About Sexual Intimacy

Nine times out of 10, efforts to talk to our teens about sexuality may flop, but on occasion, we can strike gold. Ruth, the mom in the following script, senses that the time is right to ratchet up conversations about sexual responsibility, now that her daughter, Rivka, has become increasingly more serious in her relationship with her boyfriend. Ruth approaches her daughter in a way that keeps the exchange comfortable, staying humble yet undaunted as she moves into one of the most intimate of mother-daughter conversations.

Content *(what is said)*	Process *(underlying dynamics)*
Mom (Ruth): Look, Rivka, I know this is a really touchy subject, but I have wanted to talk to you about your growing closeness with Jared.	*Mom tries a soft start-up with directness and respect.*
Rivka: (suspicious and tense) Yeah, what about it?	*Rivka senses what's ahead and tries to put Mom off.*
Mom: Well, first—I want you to know that I respect your privacy. But I feel like I need to talk to you about some things.	*Mom is not deterred by a predictable snub on this sensitive topic.*
Rivka: What?	*Rivka stays guarded.*
Mom: Since I'm sure you're growing close to him in both physical and emotional ways, I need to know whether you are thinking about the responsibilities that come with an intimate relationship.	*Mom pushes on, intent on covering her agenda to address the responsibilities of a sexually intimate relationship.*
Rivka: (groaning) Oh, no, Mom, is this going to be one of those sex talks?	*Like most teens, Rivka's first feeling about this talk is dread.*
Mom: No, this is going to be rela-	*Mom keeps her focus on the main*

Content *(what is said)*	Process *(underlying dynamics)*
tionship talk. Sex is a subtopic, as it usually should be.	*issue, which diffuses some of Rivka's testiness.*
Rivka: Mom, thanks anyway. My relationship is my business. And I'm in 10th grade—I don't need a sex talk.	*Teens think they are too sophisticated for sex information.*
Mom: Well, I do, so hang in here with me. I want to talk to you as someone who cares for you and still feels responsible for you. I don't want to be a busybody, but I do want to support you. Finding one's way through a romantic relationship is one of the most complicated things on earth—for adolescents and adults alike. I am not looking to interrogate you, really.	*Mom marches on in the way that parents must to get past the usual protests and resistance. Mom stays respectful and genuine in her care and good intentions.*
Rivka: Well, then, what are you asking for?	*Mom's gentle perseverance pays off, and Rivka softens.*
Mom: A discussion about how you are feeling.	*Mom continues carefully.*
Rivka: Don't worry, Mom, Jared and I have not had sex, if that's what you want to know.	*Rivka throws her mom a big bone to try to get her off her trail.*
Mom: Not exactly. I'm wondering how you feel about the process of growing closer.	*Mom is probably secretly thrilled and relieved, but uses the moment to go deeper.*
Rivka: Well, it's nice in most ways	*Mom's efforts are rewarded. Rivka*

Content *(what is said)*	Process *(underlying dynamics)*
and stressful in other ways.	*gives her more of an opening than she realizes.*
Mom: (quietly) What do you mean?	*This small question is the best way to keep Rivka talking.*
Rivka: I like being with him and having a boyfriend, but sometimes it's extra pressure. You know . . . am I going to disappoint him if too much of my time goes into school, soccer and my girlfriends? Do I really like him or do I just like going out with him and being linked with him? And what if we break up? Am I going to freak if one of my friends gets him instead?	*Rivka is now disarmed and gets on a roll. She freely shares a bunch of thoughts, probably not realizing how much she's letting on about this relationship.*
Mom: So you're weighing the things you like, and the doubts and worries you have.	*Mom knows the best move is active listening. She doesn't pounce on Rivka's concerns.*
Rivka: Yeah. But mainly I really like him and it's fine. I just wish I didn't feel guilty when I can't be with him as much as he wants. I feel like I hurt him and then I feel guilty.	*Rivka is able to reflect more because mom has stayed out of her way.*
Mom: Do you talk about this with him?	*Another small question invites Rivka to keep talking.*
Rivka: Well, sort of. I tell him I'm sorry a lot.	*Mom's nonjudgmental approach helps Rivka go deeper.*
Mom: It sounds hard that he's not as busy as you, and that it frustrates him. And that his frustration puts	*Mom's summary of what she has heard is a gamble because she could get it wrong, but it's close*

Content *(what is said)*	Process *(underlying dynamics)*
more pressure on you. Do you think he's more intensely attached to you than you are to him?	*enough to work.*
Rivka: Yeah. I think that we both kind of feel that. It's what creates a lot of tension. But I really want to stay with him. I do. I just wish I didn't feel so much stress about it.	*Rivka is aware of her mixed feelings, but she affirms that she wants to stay with him.*
Mom: Has deciding what you're comfortable with sexually been a source of tension?	*Another gamble, but because it's going well, Mom seizes the moment to address sexual decision-making.*
Rivka: Sort of. But I don't think either one of us is ready for that.	*Rivka shows she's on the fence about having sex.*
Mom: Do you think you know what "ready" would feel like to you?	*Mom stays right where Rivka is, whereas many parents would express an opinion or give advice at this point.*
Rivka: Well, both people would feel love and commitment for one another. They'd pretty much know that they were in a long-term situation. I don't know, Mom. Are we done yet?	*Rivka is engaging in a serious conversation about values, but indicates she has had enough.*
Mom: Doesn't readiness mean you're also ready to take responsibility for contraception?	*Mom is compelled to get to her critical point about the importance of safe sex.*
Rivka: Oh, yeah, of course, Mom. I've had enough health ed	*Rivka hints again that she's closing up shop on the talk.*

Content *(what is said)*	Process *(underlying dynamics)*
to know that.	
Mom: I said "contraception," but I mean condoms plus another method. Couples need two methods to be really safe. You've got to have condoms all the time because you never know if the person is infected.	*Mom can't resist getting out these particular points, since unsafe sex practices can be fatal, but she's running the risk of being written off as preachy.*
Rivka: (laughing) I got it. Good job, Mom! I can tell you've been reading up on the topic.	*Rivka has formally closed the conversation.*

A closer look at this exchange reveals ingredients for a successful conversation with an adolescent. When dealing with any touchy or difficult topic that might spike emotions in either person, go in with a plan. Give some forethought to your goals and know in advance what you want to cover, the process of how you're going to interact, and the pitfalls you'll need to avoid.

Ruth's overall goal is to maintain a good connection with Rivka by being supportive of her relationship with Jared and respectful of her privacy. She wants to determine whether Rivka has given much thought to what she is or isn't ready for in this romantic relationship. Ruth also needs to convey the importance of sexual responsibility and safe sex practices.

Ruth enters into the talk with a few techniques in her back pocket, and wisely exercises restraint. Any number of Rivka's attempts to steer Mom off track could have triggered a reaction, but Ruth stays gentle and deferential, persevering until she is able to get Rivka talking. Notice how Ruth stays with Rivka, picking up on what she says and nudging the conversation along, instead of catapulting ahead to conclusions or judgments. To avoid turning Rivka off—always a concern with sensitive topics—she stays small and quiet, and listens well.

In critical areas of teens' lives in which parents are highly invested—such as drugs, sex, and failure in school—they run the risk of jumping on "hot" content and becoming emotionally heated themselves. Emotionally flooded, they lose the ability to stay logical, choose the right words, and understand consequences of actions.

Hoping to avoid a bad conversation that might spoil future talks about sexuality, Ruth holds back on points she might have been dying to make. Seemingly irresistible comments like these would have quickly derailed the talk: "How in the world do you think 10th grade is too old for a sex talk?" "I'm so proud of you and Jared for restraining yourselves and saving your virginity—keep it that way." "I'm worried that Jared is stressing you out." Or, "How close are you and Jared to having sex anyway?"

Until the end of the conversation, when Rivka clearly wants out, Ruth has carefully avoided teaching or lecturing. In this way, she has built up enough "capital" that she can afford to plunge ahead and be a little pushy about the importance of using condoms plus another method for safer sex practices. Who knows when they would come this close to this topic again? Realizing it is her responsibility to get this across loud and clear, and having used masterful restraint up to now, she manages to make a critical health safety point that's likely to stick.

A List for Teens Considering Sexual Intimacy

Most of us want our teens to hold off on sexual intimacy, but we can't convince them by declaring, "You're too young to have sex." How can parents most effectively talk to their teens about readiness for sex? First, it helps to identify realistic hopes and expectations. When the time is right, we want them to appreciate sexuality as part of a healthy human identity and to be sexually well adjusted and responsible. We want sex to happen with forethought and planning, in an intimate, mature relationship with another person, and with enough awareness that they will practice safe sex. These standards set the bar pretty high, and some parents place it even higher by hoping for all this to happen only in the context of marriage.

The following list describes a set of ideal criteria that healthy, well-adjusted young people should meet before they become sexually active. The points below can be conversations starters, which allows parents to stay indirect by talking about teens in general, diffusing some of the awkwardness. Avoid personal inquiries like "Do you have this in your relationship?" Instead, get their opinions on the list; have them react to it and critique it. Using this list as a point of reference takes the pressure off a bit and may feel less intrusive to teens.

Point out the advantages of reflecting on sexual values with a clear head, separate from romantic situations. Soul searching beforehand is important, because sexual intimacy is complicated; it's hard to predict how much more intense the relationship will become and how much more vulnerable partners may feel once they begin having sex.

Teens who are considering sexual intimacy should, ideally, be responsible in these ways and have these rights in their relationships:

- They have committed to following the rules of sexual consent. Consent means actively agreeing to every advance of sexual contact. Consent can not be given under the influence.
- Even if accused of getting things heated up, they know that they have the right to make decisions about their bodies and can always say "no."
- Even if a partner pleads for sex ("If you really loved me, you would . . ." or "You owe it to me because . . ."), teens believe that it's OK to put themselves first in decisions.
- They know that being "swept away" with sex in an unplanned way is not the best way to have sex, since "unplanned" means a lack of decision making and protection, and is potentially harmful.
- Although there's a blurry line between love and sex sometimes, they're mature enough not to use sex as a way of trying to earn love.
- They are not seeking sexual intimacy as a way of dealing with personal problems or low self-esteem.
- They have the ability to talk with their partners about birth control and condoms (e.g., what method can be used—in addition to a condom— to practice safe sex).
- They have had discussions with their partners about what they would do if a pregnancy or sexually transmitted infection occurred.
- They understand that jealousy, cruelty, fighting a lot, aggressive teasing, stalking, emotional tirades, and suicidal or physical threats are all signs of an unhealthy relationship, no matter how sincere the loving talk is.
- They respect each other's feelings and differences, and realize that each partner needs to have independent friends and activities.
- Their lives are sufficiently fulfilling, so that if a break-up occurs, each person can still thrive.
- They—girls in particular—are with a partner who is roughly the same age; this is important since girls whose boyfriends are more than two years older are more likely to be exposed to alcohol, drugs, and negative consequences of their sexual activity.
- The relationship is monogamous and has been maintained over enough time to allow partners to know each other's character. No longer blinded by infatuation, the couple has faced difficulties together and resolved conflicts, and each person is confident about dealing with the emotional intensification that sex will bring.

- They are committed to avoiding having sexual relations under the influence of substances, realizing that the use of alcohol or drugs makes people more vulnerable to risky sexual encounters with unprotected sex and all of the negative consequences associated with it.

Sexual Behaviors Shock Parents

Imagine that word has leaked out about a girl and a boy in your child's middle-school class caught in the bathroom having oral sex. Taken aback, your initial reaction might be something like "Oh my God! Oral sex at age 13! What does this mean for my child?"

Whether in your child's school or reported in the media, an incident like this can be a wake-up call that you don't have a little kid anymore. Sexuality is out there, so it's best to get on with the sex education. Anything that compels parents to talk to their teens has a positive side, but when parents' anxiety flares, an infrequent incident may become exaggerated into "everyone's doing it," as if each teen is personally endangered.

Oral sex, for example, has been called "the new third base." Some teens see it as a way of being highly sexual and powerful without risking becoming pregnant. The fact that it's happening at all may be alarming, but the actual prevalence reveals that "everyone" isn't doing it, since the percentages are still low. Parents should be careful not to contribute to the buzz; doing so may actually make teens feel more comfortable joining in.

Like premarital sex in the '70s, some recent trends illustrate how behaviors that were relatively taboo in one generation can surface as the shocking new thing in the next generation. "Friends with benefits" (FWB) is a key example. FWB is an agreement to have sex with no strings attached. Whether it occurs with an existing acquaintance or with a former girlfriend or boyfriend, it tends to be prearranged, and its defining feature is that romance is strictly off limits. FWBs may limit themselves to just heavy making out or may include oral sex or intercourse.

As with many new phenomena, FWB started off among college students—busy and averse to relationships as they can be—and has pushed down to high school. Having a cute word as a description provides a certain cache and may even make it more acceptable among young people. FWB is perceived by some as an easy way to explore their sexuality without the baggage of a relationship and the chance of heartbreak when it's over. Realistically, there is often way more emotional vulnerability, confusion, and distress than anticipated. Even if the agreement was "no feelings attached," teens will still have them, and the emotional fallout can be as devastating as any romantic relationship gone awry.

An even more common phenomenon, "hooking up" can refer to a wide variety of sexual encounters, which tend to be spontaneous and involve no expectations for a relationship. Hook-ups often happen at the end of an evening, often when kids are drunk together. Teens' general impulsivity—redoubled by the lack of impulse control that goes with substance use—can result in unwanted, unsafe, and regretted sexual activity.

A generation ago, one of the big worries around sex was unwanted pregnancy. Now, because of the lethality of HIV infections and long-term negative effects of sexually transmitted infections (chlamydia, human papillomavirus, pelvic inflammatory disease, and herpes, among others), the stakes have been raised dramatically. Approximately one out of four teens has a sexually transmitted infection, but most are unaware of it because there may not be outward signs. Having sex under the influence of substances is all too common among teens. And with their judgement impaired, risks of infection and pregnancy increase. It is imperative for parents to talk to both sons and daughters about all these issues. In addition to the dangers that have been around for some time, such as date rape and unwanted pregnancy, parents need to educate themselves on new trends.

Techniques for Talking About Sex

Now and then, throughout adolescence, parents should engage in little conversations about various aspects of sexuality with their teens. Getting information across is one benefit, but an added bonus is the closeness and trust created. Compared to health-education classes, which occur on the school's schedule, parents can sense when to ramp up talks, tailoring them to the needs of the moment. For example, an important upcoming event, such as a prom, birthday, or graduation, should motivate parents to step up conversations, since big occasions often involve more risk-taking behaviors.

Different kinds of talks will occur. If you find your son at home in his bed with his girlfriend, for example, the rule violation may serve as the jumping-off point for a discussion about the consequences of breaking rules, as well as sexual responsibility. If you discover birth control pills in your daughter's drawer, the talk may take a more personal direction about health care and relationship issues. In either case, hear what the teen has to say first. Your opinions and values can follow later, but you can never replay that initial moment when they're on the hot seat. If you're calm and show a willingness to listen, they may open up in surprising ways. And we always want to let our teens know that our biggest priority is their health and safety.

Keep comments about sexuality in the context of discussions about relationships or sexual phenomena in the world, not about their sex lives specifically. Since the goal is to stimulate their thinking, try using the Socratic method: Ask open-ended questions without moralizing or weighing in. Show honest interest in their opinions and limit input mostly to facts rather than judgments. Test the waters in a relaxed way, and then if it's going well, move to weightier subjects.

Here are seven techniques for talking about sex:

1. Seize natural opportunities. Media in all forms provide daily opportunities for talks about sexuality. A news story about intimate partner violence or campus rape controversies, for example, can be an opening for talking about sexual violence or the date-rape drug (Rophynol, also called "roofies"). After seeing a provocative scene in a movie or TV show, you might say, for example, "Did it bother you that the guy was 35 and the girl was 18? What did you think?"

2. Introduce a hypothetical situation. Let's say you want to talk about condom use and safe sex. You could start a conversation with a son by saying something like, "What would you do if a friend told you he was having unprotected intercourse with a girl he didn't really know very well? Would you feel comfortable talking to him about the risk of her getting pregnant or about his risk of getting a sexually transmitted infection?" Stay in a musing mode, with comments like "Yeah, I probably wouldn't have the nerve to confront a friend unless he was a close one." And if it's going well, travel to other questions such as "How far would you go to try to keep this friend out of trouble? Would you actually buy him condoms?"

3. Practice the "please inform me" approach. With this technique, we stay humble and a little clueless, allowing them be the experts on what's going on with their generation. Let's say safe sex is again the topic. A possible opening question with a daughter might be "You've had that class on sex. Do kids make jokes about the curriculum? I know we sure did." You could try telling a funny story about a sex-ed class or you might reflect, "It's incredible what stands between life and death. You know, just a little piece of rubber. There's so much to know about safe sex. Do you think kids today are more willing to discuss some of the nitty-gritty of safe sex because of AIDS?"

4. Let your child overhear a discussion you have with a spouse or a friend. Not a calculated set-up, we simply let our teens be around and eavesdrop while we're having a heartfelt conversation about an area of concern to us. The topic can be anything—pornography, sexual harassment in the workplace, or any aspect of a love relationship. Adolescents who overhear adults deliberating over any complicated issue usually receive some food for thought.

5. Respond directly to their cues. In subtle ways, adolescents sometimes hint that they're available to talk about sexuality. This could happen, for example, in the context of negotiating new privileges. Complaining that she and her boyfriend don't get enough time alone and need more privacy, a daughter might want to renegotiate the family's bedroom open-door policy. No matter what your decision, this discussion could easily segue to a conversation about values, sexual decision making, readiness, and responsibilities.

6. Use a "third thing." Like the list earlier in this chapter, there are numerous quizzes, advice columns, and statistical reports in magazines or on the Web that can be a vehicle for a conversation. You might, for example, find a "Sex IQ" quiz on the Web, designed to determine how informed you are on various sex topics. Invite your teen to help you with one of the questions, saying, "I'm not sure about this one. What do you think?" Not only is this fun, but sex in general can be humorous, hence all the jokes. We can keep them moderately clean and still bust out some important topics with humor. A "third thing," like a quiz, can make conversations less awkward and less personal, while still stimulating awareness about sexual health and responsibility.

7. Model a healthy approach to sexuality. Parents who enjoy one another and show affection are teaching their children about the value of sexuality within a relationship. In the way that we behave toward our spouse or partner, we can demonstrate what's desirable in a relationship: connection, mutual respect, and appreciation. Our own actions can serve as one of our most powerful ways of exposing our children to the wonders of human loving.

Among our most daunting jobs as parents is helping our adolescents understand their sexual feelings, impulses, and reactions, and stay in control of their sexual choices. If we freeze up at the thought of the "sex talk," we fail to prepare our teens for someday participating in a sexual relationship that is conscious, caring, consensual, and safe.

Teens don't become sexually well adjusted by being shut off from sexual experience, or by being so free to explore sex that they are overwhelmed with more than they can integrate into positive learning experiences. Various elders in teens' lives discuss topics like careers, school, and drug use, but parents have the rare opportunity to talk about love and relationships in ways that make a deep impression. By staying calm, respectful, and supportive as we delve into these delicate issues, we get the double bonus of helping to protect our teens from the hazards of sexuality while also becoming closer to them, adding more glue to this precious relationship.

CHAPTER 12

When You're Fighting About Grades

Trouble brews in families in situations like the following:

Testing has shown that seventh-grader Ryder has solid abilities. Moreover, he attends a top-notch middle school with excellent programs and resources and an enviable student-to-teacher ratio. Despite these advantages, Ryder is pulling straight Cs. His parents are tearing out their hair because these grades will never cut it for acceptance into a selective college. Like many parents, they assume that a child with a good mind and first-rate resources should be successful in school: "My kid is smart and has all the advantages. What's wrong with demanding high achievement?" Although the teachers describe Ryder as a classic seventh-grade boy going through the tumult of adolescence, Mom and Dad conclude that he's "not motivated" and "just lazy."

Fourteen-year-old Stephen struggled to read throughout elementary school and was ultimately diagnosed with dyslexia. Except for this learning disability (LD), he tests well in other areas. Mom enlists tutors and works with the school for various accommodations, but his mediocre grades are still hard for his father to take. A successful businessman who has the same learning disability, Dad believes his son is receiving too much coddling. Having an LD himself, Dad was forced to work harder in school to overcome his LD and therein, he believes, lies the source of his success. "All this tutoring and support is just giving Stephen a way out for not doing well," Dad complains. At loggerheads, Stephen's parents are unable to agree on a plan for him.

Chloe was part of a "mean girl" group that eventually dropped her cold, and now she mopes around without any friends. This forlorn 16-year-old is forgetting to turn in assignments and study for tests, telling her parents, "I just can't get into school right now." Like many teens dealing with some extra stressor (divorce, ill parent, moving into a new neighborhood), this setback is taking a lot out of her, and it surfaces as underachievement. Unsympathetic, Chloe's parents are all over her for what they see as slacking off. "Friendship problems are a part of life," they protest. "Just buckle down and do your homework."

A teen of mixed ethnicity (African American, Caucasian, and Japanese), Keisha is constantly up against the insensitivity of her classmates in her suburban middle school, which has only 10 percent minority students in its population. "What are you?" they pester her, raising a question that jars the whole "Who am I?" struggle of adolescence. And even though she feels a pull to sit at the lunch table with other minority students, she resents that other options feel closed to her. For English class, Keisha wrote a beautiful, heartfelt paper on the confusions of racial identity, but because she had never stood out as a stellar student, the teacher accused her of plagiarism. Keisha's parents are furious with the school, accusing the teacher of racism. Out of this dreadful experience, Keisha gets the message that working hard doesn't pay off. She stops trying, and her grades plummet. Not only is there a complete breakdown in the family-school partnership, fireworks are going off at home over Keisha's bad grades.

A terrain fraught with risk for big fights, the schoolscape can become a parent-child war zone. Many parents are deeply invested in their teens' school performance—and for a very good reason. We know how much grades and education matter for a teen's future. Few college-educated parents feel comfortable when grade averages hover around C.

Understandably, many parents have high expectations, believing their teens should push aside "less important" matters (social media, gaming) to put schoolwork front and center. "So what if you're having problems with friends," a mom with a teen like Chloe might say. "This is your job. Just do it!"

We want our kids to be passionate about school, but teens report feeling both bored and stressed. With a single teacher holding forth on the implications of the Magna Carta to 30 students, many turn their attention to the clock instead of the blackboard. School is the top source of stress for teens, followed by concerns about college, and the future. Moreover, many teens don't find their classwork relevant to their lives, especially if struggling with life problems. It's not that teens lack motivation; they're plenty motivated and rarely "lazy" with activities that energize their brains, such as socializing with friends, downloading music, or pursuing new adventures.

But what about the students who have the drive to haul out the history tome, outline chapters, and commit relatively dry material to memory for the next exam? Like every other trait among teens (and humans), academic motivation and focus range from "none" to "a lot," with the complications of untidy adolescent development playing a huge role in the mix. Among the many factors prompting these high-achieving teens to get cracking, parent pressure almost always does more harm than good.

Academic performance depends on hundreds of little variables working together. Although what happens within these areas is highly complex, generally speaking, these attributes fit into four broad categories. Collectively, the "Core Four" influence how students line up.

The Core Four

Ability pertains to how individual teens process information in their brains. Although kids can develop critical thinking skills and "learn how to learn," some are born with greater capabilities and the knack for retaining, analyzing, and sequencing. Others may have issues, like a long-term diagnosed LD, or challenges that make achievement harder. Teens are "smart" in different ways; some may have perfect pitch and an ear for music, and others may have remarkable eye-hand dexterity. Still, traditional classroom work draws on a certain set of verbal and quantitative abilities, and also requires attentiveness and organization to convert these abilities into classroom success.

Personality characteristics. No matter how much intellectual horsepower a student has, other personality factors can weigh in heavily. These include characteristics such as resilience, general mood and agreeableness, level of optimism, initiative, perseverance, distractibility, and many more. A teen can have terrific academic capability, but if he is anxious, avoidant, pessimistic, and rigid, he may perform at the bottom of the class. If his parents have similar traits and are up in arms because their intelligent son isn't achieving stellar grades, he's on the road to becoming yet another smart kid who performs miserably as a student.

Emphasis on achievement. In the dream version of this quality, teens believe deeply that achievement is the path to success. Likewise, they possess an academic identity, meaning that they're invested in doing well and want to be good students because it's part of who they are. Parents may be able to influence an academic identity, but they can't force it. Studies show that parent support is crucial to achievement but the most effective means of influence is through enhancing "cognitive competence." This term refers to the extent to which students believe they possess the necessary skills to succeed in school tasks.[1] Some teens with high potential to earn straight As in a traditional academic field follow their bliss into other areas, such as the fine arts or working with their hands. Other teens feel and know that school is important, but they still aren't able to get on top of their homework, papers, and test schedules to translate their hopes into good grades. It's similar to adults wanting to value health and fitness, but falling short in efforts to eat right and exercise. A good intention is one thing; pulling it off is another. One thing is certain about academics: our kids need to know we believe in them, and they need to believe in themselves.

Social and environmental factors. Even if a student is blessed with the intellectual and emotional strengths that contribute to excelling in school, we all know that real life can get in the way. What if home life is chaotic, the neighborhood dangerous, and the school overcrowded and undersupported? Myriad factors can conspire to make students experience school and learning as unpleasant, unrewarding, and fruitless. Among them are family difficulties, poverty, shortage of role models and mentors, life stressors, and lack of opportunity.

Given the number of variables that enter into school performance—and the considerable havoc of adolescent development—why would we expect the pieces to come together perfectly? Parents often assume that it should add up nicely: a teen with a good brain + a good school system + supportive, invested parents = good school performance. But for the majority of teens, achievement is far from a straight equation.

What Kind of Student Is Your Teen?

Although individual students come in an endless variety of educational profiles, the following groupings can provide parents with the big picture of students in general and a basis for understanding their teen's school performance.

A small percentage of teens can be called **straight-shot students.** Their abilities, personality characteristics, values, and social and environmental circumstances are such that they dig into their studies, completing their homework on time, reviewing notes for tests, asking for help when needed, and going the extra distance to produce work that is above and beyond the norm. Rarely if ever are they "irresponsible." Most straight-shot students come hard-wired with just enough compulsivity and anxiety about getting good grades to keep them from slacking off on their homework to go shoot hoops. Although a good deal of "nurture" from parents can go into these students, they have likewise received gifts of "nature" from the biology they inherited.

Characteristically, straight-shot students have more of their "executive functioning" up and running. During adolescence, the brain's prefrontal cortex (our "thinking" brain) is under construction, leaving teens somewhat lacking in the executive functions that play a significant role in school achievement. These functions include emotional regulation, goal-directed persistence, flexibility, task initiation, sustained attention, and time management.

Here's how the abilities on this list might play out with 16-year-old Ian, who has a big English paper to write. Because Ian's executive functioning is working effectively, he is capable of settling down to work and creating a rough draft on time, even though he has a wicked crush on a girl in his class and has just had a fight with his brother. When his teacher critiques his thesis as too vague, he can shift directions, rethink the assignment, and revise his draft. While working on the paper over a period of two weeks, Ian hangs in there, despite other commitments competing for his time, such as household chores and a family dinner out of town at Grandma's. He even manages to complete a big chunk of the work ahead of time because he has a basketball tournament just before the deadline.

If all this sounds too good to be true, that's because only a fraction of 16-year-old boys are able to pull it off. Greater "virtues" are not what helps Ian stay focused, but rather the good fortune of his DNA and his fairly calm and organized family life. In other words, his mix of the "Core Four" provides him with the advantages to succeed in his paper.

Many teens won't have well-honed executive functioning skills until they're in their 20s, and these are exactly the abilities required to succeed starting in middle school—and more so in high school. The transitions into middle school and high school put some teens at risk for taking an academic nose dive or even dropping out, and this lag in development is one reason.

Compared to straight-shot students like Ian, by far and away, most teens are **curvy-course students,** meaning that their performance will be here and there, sprinkled with Bs and Cs and the occasional A or D. In the cases of Ryder, Stephen, Chloe, and Keisha, some variable is creating a kink in their achievement. Whether it's a situation like a teen's run-in with a biased teacher or a built-in hurdle like an LD, parents will need to be more adept in interacting with their teen, using more of the tools and advice offered in this chapter.

Because of the jumbled workings of genetic inheritance, many "straight-shot parents" end up having "curvy-course students." If Junior just happens to get Aunt Jean's problems with attention and Grandpa's depressive tendencies, his highly accomplished parents can be a nightmare for Junior when they badger him about his average grades.

How easy it is to misjudge an energetic teen boy who won't revise his paper even though it could hike up his grade, or the scatterbrained girl who gives her homework short shrift, preferring to hang out at the mall. These behaviors would aggravate the most understanding parent because, as teens bobble around in their own little bubbles of concerns, we know about the impact of those C's, D's and F's. Nevertheless, positive attitudes and encouragement of curvy-course students from parents remains critical. As their brains mature and their executive functions lock in at different points in time, the rubber may hit the road and school may finally become a priority.

Squeaker students, who show little effort and are barely passing in school, present an even greater challenge for parents. These teens often do better in alternative school programs with a less conventional teaching approach, a lower student-to-teacher ratio, and more day-to-day accountability. Parents of squeaker students will need to mobilize more resources to keep their teens from bottoming out of the school system. Lectures may be on the tip of the tongue, and power struggles can lurk at each impasse. Parents will probably have to work extra hard to avoid these pitfalls while revamping school and home life to help squeakers get more on course.

At the clinical end of the spectrum are **failing students,** who are in deep trouble in the school system and probably in the rest of their lives as well. School failure is often accompanied by these behaviors: excessive absenteeism, lack of connection with the school, ongoing discipline problems at school, limited goals for the future, and a belief that school is "worthless and stupid and irrelevant." If parents see these behaviors taking root, they should get professional help immediately.

Given the profound importance of education, parents shouldn't hesitate to pursue an assessment, ideally long before their student descends into failure. Gone are the days when parents needed to worry that professional help would make their kids feel bad. It's the 21st century and we all need help sometimes!

Family Story: A Lackadaisical Student Piles on the Excuses

Fifteen-year-old Suri is throwing her mom and dad for a loop. Experience shows that with a little effort she can do very well, but throughout middle school she was usually too wrapped up in her world of friends to give a hoot about grades. During eighth grade, this outgoing teen had a pattern of completing assignments at the eleventh hour or not turning them in at all, earning her share of Cs—and an occasional D.

With high school looming and serious concerns about Suri's underachievement, Mom and Dad call a family meeting at the end of the summer to establish rules for screen use and homework hours for ninth grade. A teen who could talk her way out of any jam, Suri implores her parents for a chance to improve her grades on her own, begging them, "Just trust me. I really want to do better."

Despite Suri's recent problematic track record and the lack of a specific plan for turning her performance around, Mom and Dad relents, warning her, "We need to see a 3.0 GPA or else."

Guess what happens when the first ninth-grade progress report arrives? The two scripts below illustrate diverse approaches by two different dads, each handling their "Suris." Dad no. 1, Roger, charges at the problem and gets nowhere, while dad no. 2, Daniel, remains calm, finessing the situation and ultimately reaching an agreement that places some limits on his sociable daughter.

Suri and Roger: accusatory and reactive

Content *(what is said)*	Process *(underlying dynamics)*
Dad (Roger): Suri, I just saw your progress report. I couldn't believe my eyes—two D's and a C! This is a disaster. What do you have to say for yourself?	*Although this is a natural way for an anxious and concerned parent to feel, it is negative and unlikely to yield a productive conversation.*
Suri: They are only midterm grades—it's because they didn't have all my homework yet and a couple of stupid little tests. Chill, Dad. You should see how red your face is.	*Like a law of physics, when one party is perceived as exaggerating, the other party is likely to minimize in order to tilt the emotional balance.*
Dad: You have manipulated us again. When we tried to set you up with a homework plan last summer, you begged to "handle it yourself." Now you're blowing your GPA the second you hit high school. I feel taken for a sucker. You are being totally irresponsible, just like you were all through eighth grade.	*Roger is frustrated that he trusted Suri to change her pattern of procrastination. Parents who feel ineffective or hoodwinked often accuse the teen of manipulation. In actuality, when these teens say they can "handle it," they're simply trying to get their parents off their back. Apparently, that part worked, but the grades are still suffering.*
Suri: You're not listening. I'll get my homework in and then it'll be fine. And those tests were ridiculous.	*Sometimes when teens present their edited stories, stitched together to seem compelling, we feel*

Content *(what is said)*	Process *(underlying dynamics)*
The Spanish teacher admitted the entire curve was off, so everybody made terrible grades. Don't worry, I'll fix it.	*manipulated. The problem is that they believe what they're saying, even if we don't.*
Dad: I can't believe you are repeating the same hogwash as last year. Do you think I'm an idiot? Listen, young lady, the jig is up. We are taking away your cell phone until we see all A's and B's. And forget weekend fun—you're grounded. We've had it with your slacking off.	*When parents feel "taken for a sucker," they sometimes react swiftly with punitive limits to attempt a big intervention with the hopes for big results. Instead, the goal should be organizing a system with Suri's input so that she has buy-in on a plan to improve her grades.*
Suri: Dad, I told you I could fix this. How can you take everything I care about away from me? Do you really think that is going to work? I'll be so mad and deranged, I'll never get anything done. You just want me to be miserable because I can't be as perfect as you want me to be.	*Most cool-headed people could have predicted this backfire effect, but we can also appreciate the hot-headed impulse to lay down the law with an unruly child. Suri's last slam reveals another piece of her academic story.*

Here is a calmer approach to the same situation with a different dad.

Suri and Daniel: calm, careful, and skillful

Content *(what is said)*	Process *(underlying dynamics)*
Dad (Daniel): So, we agreed last summer that if the progress report was not all B's or above that we would institute more formal homework rules. Do you want to propose some, or should I?	*Daniel may have felt as upset as Roger had, but he has cooled off and planned his approach carefully in hopes of enlisting Suri's cooperation.*

Content *(what is said)*	Process *(underlying dynamics)*
Suri: Dad, the grades look worse than they are. I didn't have all my homework in. The Spanish teacher said she might redo the curve because so many kids flunked the midterm.	*Suri really believes her story, even though a parent may hear it as "blah, blah, blah." She will try anything to avoid parental surveillance.*
Dad: A deal is a deal, and I told you to be prepared to propose some ideas, since I imagine you will like yours better than you'll like your parents'.	*Daniel knows better than to react to Suri's excuses. He sticks to the goal of trying to steer Suri toward solving her own problems. Any solution she comes up with stands a better chance of working than something he dictates.*
Suri: Dad, whatever you do, don't take my cell away. I know you threatened that last summer, but that would kill me. I'm not kidding. Homework is torture without some contact with the world. Plus, my friends and I help each other with homework with FaceTime.	*Suri sounds like one of those teens who believe that a cell phone is her lifeline, feel that homework is a torment and that mixing the two is a way to make it tolerable. At least Daniel has her thinking about the new policy.*
Dad: OK, so your cell and contact with your friends is incredibly important. And homework is an awful experience for you, right?	*One of the hardest communication rules for parents to learn is that empathy costs nothing, benefits our goal of engendering cooperation greatly, and doesn't mean we agree with anything.*
Suri: Right. But we need a plan where I keep my cell phone.	*Notice that she's now participating in the planning process and using "we."*
Dad: So, instead of no cell phone at all, what if we shut off contact with friends for a 90-minute	*Dad's warning last summer about terminating her cell phone privilege makes this plan look*

Content *(what is said)*	Process *(underlying dynamics)*
homework session after dinner?	*relatively benign.*
Suri: Oh, God, I'll hate it, but it's better than losing it the whole night. Fine. It will feel like jail time. I hope you know that.	*Suri is barely tolerating this impingement, but Daniel's cooperative approach has paid off.*

A striking difference exists between the two dads' tactics and the outcomes. Running at the problem like a bull, Roger makes all the mistakes of a parent who is anxious about his daughter ruining her GPA and college options. Frustrated by his daughter's blasé and defensive attitude, he hits the roof when Suri falls short of last summer's promise.

Although his feelings are valid, Roger's methods are ineffective. Since he imposes a new policy on Suri without any input from her and in a punitive way, his parenting approach can be considered authoritarian, an unproductive parenting style characterized by a lot of control, little warmth, and ineffective communication. Roger is all accusation and no understanding, a combination that usually backfires. In fact, Suri tells him as much. Now, instead of Suri assuming increased responsibility for her grades, she can point the finger at "dictator dad" as a handy excuse for continued coasting.

By contrast, Daniel shows how to advance skillfully through the same situation with more successful results. Daniel realizes that unless Suri buys into the new program, it will lead nowhere. He also appreciates that her emotional brain experiences homework as torture. Rather than arguing about the drama of her comment, he negotiates a policy that will help her cope with some parameters for dreaded homework time.

Parents can talk until they're blue in the face about the importance of grades for college selection and opportunities ahead. As compelling as that is to most adults, teens like Suri don't think realistically about the future. Wisely, Daniel skips the conversational merry-go-round, focusing instead on solving the problem.

Suri's statements "I'll handle it" and "I'm fixing it" are not so much lies as magical thinking. In other words, while still hating homework and studying, she has no strategies for change, believing instead that she will somehow— cross your fingers!—pull herself out of the hole. Teens are bundles of contradictions, yet rarely do they have insight into them. Only the most naïve parents waste energy lecturing a teen about contradicting herself. Curvy-course students rarely offer clear explanations for why their academics are on tilt, because the issues are far more complex than they can fully articulate. Likewise, teens are never going to agree happily with a parent's position that since the teen has blown it, the parent has a right to feel upset, betrayed, or worried for them. A shame-based approach focusing on the parent's negative feelings about poor grades just plain doesn't work.

Academic success for Suri will be more complicated than just implementing a study hall and turning over her cell phone. She'll still be able to communicate with friends and fritter away her homework time using her laptop. But Daniel has established a first step toward collaborating with Suri on her study habits, and they can work together on monitoring homework completion as the next step. As minimal as the 90-minute cell phone yank may seem, it's a step in the right direction and she's now on board. Once Suri and her parents are on the same team, they can work toward agreeing on other steps, described in the next section.

Help on the Home Front for Disappointing Grades

In a perfect world, our teens would seize their educational opportunities and develop the study habits needed to earn excellent grades, but these behaviors belong to the small percentage of straight-shot students. Parents can hold out a beacon for academic success, but they should realize that most teens' report cards will include a mix of B's and C's.

What are some ways that parents can lend a hand (or more accurately, part of their brain) to their curvy-course or squeaker students? Keep in mind that we don't intervene when the first low grade is earned, but rather when grades as a whole are slipping.

Here are some recommendations:

Don't make it worse. Criticizing, lecturing, and threatening are among the most pervasive yet least effective parental reactions to teens' grade slumps. Parents' feelings may be valid, but the question remains: Can you affect your teen's performance positively with more words, focus, and pressure? Receiving poor grades is one of those hot-button areas. When disappointing reports roll in, put yourself on pause until you're calm and then choose your approach strategically.

Keep a positive relationship. Some parents inadvertently risk their relationship with their teen—adopting punishing, coercive, and other negative tactics—for the idea that they can do something to raise grades, but they'll fail miserably unless the teen is motivated. Teens and parents need to be aligned. With a good relationship and mostly positive interactions, parents maintain influence, one of the most effective tools in the parent toolbox.

Link homework and good grades to social freedoms or—temporarily—to enticing perks. Some teens benefit from a system wherein parents tie completion of homework to social privileges on weekends, saying, "First you do your homework, then you have your free time."

Other families devise a tangible reward system, but using a "carrot" to encourage kids has a downside, because students who are externally motivated tend to let down over time. Rewards stimulate some teens, because the positive "goody" can override the negative feeling of tackling homework. Nevertheless, hold off on this approach until grades are truly sliding, and any perk should be a temporary benefit that is phased out when the teen starts to experience success. Ideally, the internal rewards of doing well should take precedence over external motivators.

Organize the home turf. When a teen's school performance is deteriorating, educators unanimously agree that revamping study habits can make all the difference. Teens need independence and room to be responsible for their assignments and grades, but many also need a structure to support their success. Given the complexity of their lives and their lapses in executive functioning, some teens may need their parents' help in planning, organizing, and persisting. The challenge for parents is finding a balance—intruding as little as possible while also helping a disorganized teenager manage his social, athletic, and otherwise busy life to include a time and place for concentrating on schoolwork.

Below are some steps that teens and parents can agree on for retooling study habits when teens' grades are sliding:

- Decide on a block of time for home study hall. The more problematic the homework habits, the more helpful it will be to create a cut-and-dried study period. This can range from 30 minutes to two hours, depending on grade level and school demands. Don't budge. Even if the teen says his homework is done, this period can be used for reading. The biggest sabotage of homework time is media.

- Limit access to media. Today's wired world leaves students with little undiluted time for concentrating and thinking deeply and creatively. Teens claim to be able to watch YouTube, track social media sites, answer the phone, and do homework simultaneously, but the research results are in: Multi-tasking effectiveness is a fantasy for adults and more so for teens. If you need to negotiate with your teen, consider allowing music, because the positive emotions of music sometimes help teenagers better tolerate studying.

• Figure out the best location. Teens may need to be separated from siblings, distractions, or whatever media device is undermining homework. Sometimes a comfortable common space, such as a kitchen in the evening, can work better than an isolated room.

• Determine whether parent "coaching" will be effective. Ideally, parents should nudge teens toward self-reliance, but many curvy-course students are overwhelmed by big assignments and need help breaking them down into doable chunks with short, manageable deadlines. A whiteboard can be a fabulous aid for this. If teens agree, parents can help set up schedules and may even hang out with teens as they research subjects and plan their approach. This kind of scaffolding should be temporary, since the goal is to pull it away and leave teens standing independently. When teens with slumping grades resist parent coaching, consider hiring a tutor.

• Consult with teachers or school counselors, who may have additional ideas and insights into the problem. Form a partnership with the school that will help your teen improve her performance and assume responsibility for achievement.

Stressed out over disappointing grades, parents can become zealous about overhauling old habits in one fell swoop, but it's better to work gingerly with teens. Turnarounds take patience, persistence, a positive attitude, and, mostly, time.

Seven Top Tips for Boosting School Achievement

One of today's little secrets: Teens can become dependent on parents to the point that they fear they can't make the grade without parental help. Some well-meaning parents put their teens' papers into a word-processing program's editing mode, and all the teen has to do is "accept changes." When parents become a crutch, teens feel like a sham, and this dependence whittles away at their self-esteem, because they know they're not doing the work themselves. No one feels good, but who wants to give it up and risk a bad grade?

Teens need to be given the freedom to experience the feelings of doing well on their own. Still, parents' hands are far from tied in what they can legitimately do to stimulate engagement in school work. The following information is a synthesis of top tips from educational pros.

1. Be an authoritative parent. Research shows that academically motivated teens come from families in which parents have high expectations and also encourage independence. An authoritative parenting style has been linked to achievement motivation.[2] As one might expect, parenting that is warm, firm, and fair works better than parenting that is punitive, harsh or overly strict (authoritarian), or detached or inept (permissive). With healthier beliefs about achievement and a positive value on learning, authoritative parents are neither overcontrolling perfectionists nor hands off and disengaged. Likewise, they tend to be involved with the school, interacting effectively with teachers.

2. Become a cheerleader. While overpraising has its own problems, kids need to feel as if their parents "have their back" in school and in life. A parent's crucial role in a teen's education is to support, encourage, ignore minor slippages, and keep a 5–1 ratio of positive to negative interactions. Nothing is more exasperating than when a teen with a good brain does poorly in school, but too much worrying often leads parents to believe, "It's my responsibility to make sure my child succeeds in school." Likewise, parents can overidentify with their teen, believing that poor grades reflect badly on them and their parenting. These misconceptions can translate into thoughtless statements that actually undermine performance, such as:

It's not that I care about grades—I just hate to see you throw away your potential.

I just know you'd be happier if you got good grades, because you'll be able to get into a better college and then get a better job.

I thought you wanted to improve your grades! Why are you always glued to your phone?

I don't understand why I'm paying all this money for tutoring, because you're still getting bad grades.

If you don't bring those grades up, you'll be grounded until they improve!

You're just lazy.

Your report card was great, but what's with this B?

Avoid these kinds of statements like the plague, since we now know definitively that pressuring kids in school does damage. Recent studies in suburban America show the harm of a preoccupied focus on grades. Among affluent, advantaged children, academic pressure is correlated to depression, anxiety, substance use, and alienation from parents.[3]

3. Adopt the right attitude toward achievement. Let's say that you have a teen who does well in school. Should you encourage her by continually telling her that she's smart? Although some 85 percent of parents say "yes," major research begs to differ.[4] This type of remark contributes to a "fixed mind-set" about intelligence. Thirty years of research shows that students who believe their ability is fixed (that is, it's a "given," not subject to change) don't try as hard as those who believe their abilities are malleable. We now know that intelligence is far more changeable than once believed. When students with a fixed mind-set experience a failure, they're quicker to assume they're not very smart after all.

Instead of praising kids for being "smart," praise them for being "good learners," remarking on the processes they use for achieving: working hard, concentrating, rallying after a setback, getting help when they're struggling, or asking teachers to clarify assignments. Show interest in the way they think, placing a value on expanding skills and knowledge. This approach has a positive effect on academic confidence, which in turn impacts motivation. Kids who are confident in their ability to learn tend to hang in there when the going gets tough.

4. Be aware of the "panther in the backpack." Teens can have incredibly negative emotions about schoolwork: fear of failure, resentment about not being as smart as other kids, worry that even one's best effort won't be good enough—not to mention sheer dread of the workload. It's no different from all the things we adults dread and avoid, such as cleaning the garage, doing the taxes, or talking about difficult topics with loved ones. And like teens, we invent our own "cop-out" statements to postpone what we dread.

Here's the rub: Teens are rarely able to articulate their deep anxiety about schoolwork. Within all procrastinators lies some kind of anxiety, but it's beyond them to say, in essence, "I see a panther when I see my backpack," even though their emotional brains might register their pile of homework as predatory. Stress is a toxin to learning. Hormones are released; the brain seizes up; and neural circuits can't process academic information or retrieve memories.[5] Teens compartmentalize their negative feelings in a little box that's inaccessible to parents. All we notice is the teenager postponing or neglecting homework. We won't have a clue that anxiety is the reason for their avoidance. When they shrug indifferently and say, "I don't have any homework," or "I'll do it later," we react with our own anxiety to the carelessness we perceive in our teen. In response, the teen compartmentalizes even more. Parents need to realize that there's more to procrastination than meets the eye.

Anxiety is a double-edged sword: A certain amount of it can energize, make us alert, and help us stay focused, but too much can lead to "fight, flight, or freeze" reactions and block access to the executive functions needed to tackle tests or homework assignments. Anxious, perfectionist parents can make things worse, because negative emotions about schoolwork can be flooding the teenager from within and without. Stress reduction techniques such as meditation, exercise, sleep, play, social outlets, and time in nature can improve this state of affairs. Parents can help by attending to their angst so that they don't infuse the teen with their own stress.

5. Realize that academic thriving involves the whole child. Support the various building blocks of your teen's life: home, school, extracurricular activities, and friendships. Instead of fixating on grades, grades, grades, keep your eye on the big picture of what improves your teen overall, because this will likely perk up their school performance. Starting with middle school, create a family policy of having your teen participate in sports and school-based extracurricular activities. Zero activity should not be an option, given the research linking school connectedness to school success.

Attend school functions and be involved in what happens there. When teens complain or blame teachers for difficulties, work to solve problems with your teen and hold off on criticizing the school. Although parents will need to jump in if there is a clear problem of bullying, teacher abuse, or disciplinary injustice, work with the school, not against it.

Having friends who make good grades and aspire to college can enhance a teen's achievement. Nevertheless, if your teen has fallen into a non-academic peer group, instead of agonizing about "bad peers," focus on a balanced routine of extracurricular activities, schoolwork, family dinners, and responsibilities, and very little socializing on weeknights. This kind of regime will automatically keep teens busy and not completely surrendered to a peer culture.

6. Counteract educational gender stereotyping. Because each of the sexes has certain advantages and disadvantages in school, parents should be on the lookout for ways to advocate for both daughters and sons. Girls' brains mature earlier, setting them up to read and write better, and providing them with more developed executive-functioning abilities. Also, girls are socialized to behave better in all the ways that schooling requires. But there's a definite downside. Because girls are sometimes not encouraged to take advanced math, science, and computer courses—and may pick up on the "boys only" messages in these future careers—parents may need to spur them on.

Although boys are nudged to take the "harder" sciences, their brain development is two years behind their female classmates. This lag, together with their boisterous ways, means boys are more likely to be diagnosed with behavior, learning, and attention disorders. When boys get into trouble, they often just shut down, or they cover their shame with defiance, adding to the misunderstanding. Parents and educators alike can benefit from reading more about boys' emotional development to understand what a struggle it is for some boys to sit in class all day or to deal with vulnerable feelings.

7. Consider other secrets to success. Anything that increases a teen's happiness quotient, self-esteem, and confidence can enhance school achievement. Here are other ways to do just that.

• Plan summers strategically. Although teens may scream for their rights to "hang out," a surplus of free time can be trouble. In middle-school years, camp can be just the ticket. Summer activities should not be about the college résumé. Instead, consider what else would enhance your teen's development and expose her to new horizons: employment, being out in nature, public service, or visiting a relative in another part of the country to work on a farm, for example. Unless a teen has a significant problem or disability, or a consultant has made a persuasive case, summer tutoring won't automatically result in improved school performance, especially if the teen isn't on board.

• Help your teen think about career options—maybe through a part-time job, internship, informational interview, "shadow" day in a job setting, or conversations with your friends about their careers.

• Encourage volunteering. Even if your teen is employed, helping others who are less fortunate or being exposed to the nonprofit world opens up valuable new perspectives on life.

• Consider carefully the pros and cons of paid work. Advantages can include developing a work ethic, learning about one's interests, overcoming shyness with adults, and enhanced self-esteem. The cons typically include compromised time for family, friends, and academics. To understand the consequences of teenage work, parents need to think about the experiences their teens will have while working — the quantity as well as the quality of work, plus their teen's particular needs, academic promise, and motivations to work.[6] For some teens, work can be a springboard to a job after high school, while in other circumstances, the teen may just want money to squander on junk food, alcohol, and stuff.

The bottom line is: Don't ever give up on championing your teen's education. Progress in school can be a long and winding road for curvy-course or squeaker students, since many are waylaid and misunderstood in the school setting. Nonetheless, all the research points to clear advantages to persevering in the educational journey.

What Matters More Than the Numbers Game

When a teen receives acceptance into an elite college, parents sometimes congratulate themselves for being "good parents," as if they deserve more credit than the moms and dads who committed themselves to the hard work of supporting and encouraging other kinds of students. What a misassumption it is to believe that straight-shot students are more virtuous or promising individuals!

Top achievers in high school often do become top achievers in college, but with brain maturation and personal development, many curvy-course students become star performers in college, careers, and life. Even though lackluster students can outdo school-smart kids in later life, we overlook this phenomenon and fall back on numbers (GPA, SAT scores, class rankings).

During the launching process from high school to college, parents' perspectives can become skewed by anxiety and the unknowns that lie ahead. The college admissions frenzy and concerns that "it's harder than ever to get into a good school" can distort parents' beliefs and drive them to become preoccupied with grades. First, there is a problem with the word "good."

Eighty percent of applications go to 20 percent of the colleges, leaving plenty of excellent schools that accept most of their applicants. Second, where a teen attends college does not predict occupational success as much as what he does with that experience and his degree of engagement.[7]

Smart parents focus on their relationship with their teen and the broader range of developing characteristics that actually do set teens up for academic, occupational, and personal success. Intellectual interest is only one of a whole set of strengths that go into a winning mix. Extensive research has shown how important social and emotional learning (SEL) can be in enhancing a students' academic performance.[8]

Parents should to keep a wide-open lens when thinking about all of the qualities in a child's character that need to be developed for a successful launch to college. The following is a list of such qualities, based largely on studies in emotional intelligence.

The Big 10 Characteristics of a Successful Teen[9]

1. Motivation and drive
2. Practical reasoning and judgment
3. Moral attentiveness and character
4. Emotional awareness
5. Healthy habits
6. Self-control and emotional management
7. Social skills and an ability to maintain quality relationships
8. Communication skills
9. Intellectual interests and abilities
10. Spirituality/religious faith

Whenever you become discouraged about your teen's grades, shift some of your attention to this list and think of what you can do to adjust, leverage, or bolster qualities that make for personal success. Shine the light on your teen's winning qualities. Although harder to measure than a test score, these 10 characteristics woven together over time explain the thriving of young adults far better than any numbers.

———————————

As in other areas of teen development, parents sometimes struggle with whether to focus less or more on a teen's school progress. The solution usually lies somewhere in the middle and in working with a teen's unique mix of abilities, personality characteristics, values, and circumstances. If grades are in a slump, try to understand why. Broaden your view to include adjustments in home study habits, attention to the teen-parent relationship, and a shoring up of "Big 10" qualities.

Teens feel harassed by parents who hover over their school life. As important as investing in a teen's school performance is, stressing out does no good and may even hurt, since it limits the broader view of a teen and what else is going on in his life. No parent wants their relationship with their teen to devolve into a distant one about which the teen says, "All my parent cares about is grades."

As tricky as the "sex talk," the "grade talk" that follows a disappointing school report can easily go sideways. Three all-too-common elements of the "grade talk" include: reminding the teen of the importance of school, emphasizing their high potential (which is supposed to be a compliment), and admonishing them to be more motivated and responsible. Equally predictable, teen responses include the hanging head, the rolling eyeballs, the lame excuses, or the hostile and defensive retorts. Teens are usually incapable of unpacking all the emotions and reasons for unsatisfactory schoolwork. It's up to us to add up what we can discern from our teen's explanation, our own insights, and feedback from teachers, and then make a plan, with input from the teen. This is an area in which a little less talk and a little more very thoughtful action pay off.

And don't forget to model a love for learning and the life of the mind. Teens may not show their intellectual leanings consistently during the jumbled years of adolescence, but parents are often impressed by how their own reading and studying habits, which they've demonstrated and gently encouraged, take hold in their children later on.

CHAPTER 13

When You Catch Your Teen With Alcohol or Drugs

Today's average teen is bombarded by anti-substance-use messages in the media: testimonials of hip kids choosing not to drink, warnings linking cigarette smoking to horrible illnesses if not death, and portrayals of the dire consequences of drinking and driving. Yet, despite those public-health campaigns, in 15 minutes of channel surfing, teens are inundated with dozens of images glamorizing smoking and showing the fun of drinking and socializing. A parade of celebrities shows various ways that alcohol, drugs, and cigarettes (together called "substance" use) are desirable, cool, and image enhancing.

Teens receive inconsistent messages in their daily lives. On the same day, one teen discovered with a beer might be expelled from school, while another gets a slap on the wrist from a police officer or a wink and a nod from a parent.

Mixed messages prevail, from idealized (and for most teens, unrealistic) expectations that a teen should "just say no" to ominous (and for most teens, exaggerated) warnings that substance addiction and hard-drug abuse can result from even a little experimentation. Because patterns of substance use among teens are far more complex than either of these positions suggests, neither message really reaches teenagers.

As parents, we've been told to convey clear expectations to our teens about alcohol, drugs, and cigarettes, but we're living in a world full of contradictions and messages that ping-pong between extremes. No wonder many parents fumble when trying to talk to their teens about substance use and create a realistic family policy.

Many parents find themselves trying to reconcile their hopes that their teens will steer clear of substances with the knowledge that they probably won't. Although there's no easy solution, when a parent's approach is based in reality—recognizing and straddling the numerous contradictions—that parent comes across as more credible, improving the odds that teens will listen better to critical messages about safety and health.

Why Risk Is a Teen's Middle Name

There's no denying it: Compared to young children and adults, teenagers engage in more risky behavior. Some risk taking is healthy, a way for teens to grow, learn, stretch in new directions, and accept new challenges; for example, when they run for a school office, start to learn a new musical instrument, or join the mountaineering club. But teens are also more likely than adults to drive recklessly, use illicit substances, have unprotected sex, and participate in illegal activities. To their benefit and to their peril, there's a lot more experimenting during adolescence.

By around age 15, teens have abilities similar to those of adults for understanding and assessing risk in a "cold" logic situation, but in highly arousing, real-life situations, teens' reasoning can falter. This shortcoming is tied into their changing biology. By their very nature, teens are more drawn to novelty, more susceptible to sensation seeking, and less able to self-regulate; a combination that leads them to accept risks, for better or worse.

In the normal range of negative risk taking (meaning most teens will do them) are behaviors such as breaking rules, driving unsafely, flirting with potential dangers, and in this same category, experimenting with substances. As much as we wish otherwise, these hazardous yet exciting behaviors are part of what defines adolescence.

Typically, parents have their eyes out for alcohol, but there's every reason to be equally if not more alarmed about teens getting hooked on cigarettes. Nicotine use is related to cancer, heart disease, lung disease, and greater susceptibility to disease in general, with around 480,000 people dying of tobacco-related illnesses in the United States every year. About 3,200 kids take up smoking daily. Teens who become occasional smokers can progress to daily smoking, putting them on the road to addiction.

Teens are more likely than adults to become addicted to nicotine; moreover, teens become addicted more quickly. From the successful lawsuits against the tobacco companies in the 1990s, we learned that teens were being specifically targeted in advertising efforts. Tobacco companies were banking on the fact that most lifetime smokers (80 percent of them) begin using cigarettes before the age of 18. If smoking doesn't become a habit before 18, getting hooked for life is less likely.

Results from the 2015 National Youth Risk Behavior Survey revealed that even though cigarette smoking among high schoolers has dropped to the lowest levels since the survey began in 1991, the use of e-cigarettes among teens is concerning and on the rise.[1] Always game for trying new things, teens are especially vulnerable to the lure of candy-flavored nicotine and vaporizers that look like pens, mascara, and lipstick.

This same survey found that 42 percent of high schoolers who drive admit to texting or emailing while driving. The dangers of handling a phone while driving has been statistically equated with driving while intoxicated. And parents who are guilty of the same behaviors are hardly good models for their teens. One study conducted in the emergency department of a hospital found that two-thirds of parents admitted to driving while talking on the cells with children in the car and one-third admitted to texting.[2] Let's face it—all humans are susceptible to the dopamine-rich rewards of nicotine and technology use, but teens even more so.

Another major survey of adolescents called "Monitoring the Future" and funded by the National Institutes of Health issued their results in 2016 on teen substance use, revealing news both good and bad.[3] The good news is that the use of alcohol, marijuana, prescription medications, and illicit substances declined in 2016. Furthermore, the use of drugs among eighth-graders was at its lowest in decades. Nonetheless, high school seniors surveyed used cannabis in some form at least once within the last month. The big concern is the 6 percent reporting daily use. Thirty-seven percent of seniors reported that they had gotten drunk at least once during the last year, which is down from a peak of 53 percent in 2001. While the use of painkillers is also down in high schoolers, the opiate addiction crisis among adults keeps us all wary of where this trend is headed.

As alarming as the facts and figures are, they tell us little about whether any individual teen's life will be harmed in the long run by experimenting with substances. If a teen starts using substances in middle school, drinks heavily, binges, or shows any problematic pattern of use, he's obviously at risk, and parents need to take strong measures to intervene and get a specialist on board. The picture is less clear for the experimenters. A percentage of kids who try alcohol and other drugs will, indeed, have the biological make-up and the risk factors that lead to dependency (for example, problems with school, behavioral compliance, or motivation). However, many teens who toy with substances never move on to regular or heavy use.

Experimenting with substances is not altogether negative. It's one of the paradoxes of adolescence that while alcohol and drug use negatively impact teens' brains, this experience itself also teaches them about risk. Neuroscientists point out that teens show more activity in their memory centers than adults when they are taking risks in lab experiments, leading to speculation that learning is likewise occurring. If teens never go to a party, how are they supposed to learn how to moderate and manage themselves in those situations? Nonetheless, figuring out how keep substance use minimized and safe is one of the biggest challenges for families during the teen years.

Parents take stock of a variety of typical adolescent behaviors—like teens' push for independence or their budding sexuality—and we likewise need to ask ourselves, "How am I going to deal with substance use?" Most teens are asking themselves this same question! Some adolescent health specialists see substance use as inextricably tied into teenage life these days, forming a part of a teen's identity, values, and self-definition.

A black-and-white approach to substances (zero tolerance!) boxes parents in. The minute teens sip beer with friends, they become "bad," and we become restricted in our parenting options by our own rigid stance. Substance use is never acceptable, but we still want to stay connected with our teens when they take risks that make us uncomfortable. We need to move in and work with them, supervising more closely and limiting opportunities for getting into trouble, while also giving them room to have a social life. A realistic approach to teen substance use looks hard at the data to see that "eliminating" may not be in the cards. Safety, health, and harm reduction become our goals.

The Teen Brain and Substances: A Unique and Scary Brew

Substance abuse is obviously detrimental to all humans, but this is particularly true for teens, because their biology renders them uniquely vulnerable.

Heavy drinking interferes with the encoding of new memories. A neurotransmitter called glutamate, which aids in learning and storing new memories, is affected by alcohol. No wonder people don't remember anything the morning after a big alcohol bash. The effect is especially damaging for adolescent brains, which are undergoing the "pruning and blossoming" of new neural pathways; glutamate helps this wiring process. Extensive alcohol use leads to glutamate dysfunction, which leads to problems with learning and memory.

On top of harmful effects on memory and learning, when teens use alcohol, their young brains are being primed to find it pleasant, rewarding, and necessary for well-being. Here's how: Like other drugs, alcohol and nicotine stimulate the release of the neurotransmitter dopamine. (Neurotransmitters are chemicals that send messages between neurons.) Got dopamine? Then you've got the sense of pleasure, and as we all know, pleasure sometimes confers benefits and sometimes gets us into trouble. Dopamine is part of the human body's system for survival. The association of food and sex with pleasure and the drive to "do it again" helps to ensure that we neither starve nor become extinct as a species. Mind- and mood-altering substances associated with pleasure seeking (sometimes connected to religious or tribal rituals) have been recorded as far back as the beginning of recorded history. By generating a memory for a source of pleasure, dopamine teaches the brain what it wants and then creates a need to repeat the behavior to feel the reward again, regardless of whether it's good for you.

Different people struggle with different guilty pleasures or bad habits. When people are thinking straight, their rational brains may remind them to pull back on bad habits (excess drinking, eating junk food, having casual sex, overspending, watching too much TV), overriding the impulse to seek gratification again. Between their immature impulse-control centers and their extra sensitivity to dopamine, teens are primed for risk-taking.

As widely observed, something happens to teens in the presence of peers. A common quip is that the average IQ level of a bunch of teens drops by 10 points for every friend that is added to the group. Whether it pertains to trying pot or an impetuous shoplift, when teens are around each other they are more susceptible to the sway of their similarly risk-prone peers. Why is this so?

Many parents continue to use the phrase "peer pressure" even though most risky behaviors happen without any "pressure" per se. While it's true that they're with peers and there is definitely influence, the interaction is more complex. We know that, in general, groups of people take more risks together than individuals do alone. This phenomenon is called the "risky shift," meaning that once the behavior gets rolling, others are more likely to go along with it.

Contagion of this sort is even more pronounced for groups of younger teens (ages 12–14). The remodeling of the brain during early adolescence makes the release of dopamine that accompanies risk taking even more rewarding and pleasurable while in the presence of peers. It's not fully understood how dopamine works in the emotional brain; suffice it to say that because of the way dopamine and arousal around peers mingle in the teen brain, the mix of peers with substances or other risky and exciting ventures creates one big pleasure high.[4]

This phenomenon has a huge range, depending on the teen and the circumstances. Depending largely on temperament, some kids may actually shy away from harmful peer situations. A low level of increased excitement can be subtle and easily managed, while at other times—and with particular teens—it can lead to off-the-wall risk taking and reckless behavior.

With the greater self-regulation that accompanies brain development in the twenties, risk taking declines, but during the teen years, the need for parental vigilance takes on new dimensions.

Good Moves for Sticky Situations

Our run-ins with teens over small annoyances—the smirk, the self-centeredness, the inconsistent follow-through—can pale in comparison to dealing with substance use. Reeling from the shock that "my teen" is the one caught with the gin, parents can become anxious, flummoxed, and overwhelmed, thinking extreme thoughts: Who has my teen become? Do I even know her anymore? Is she endangered? Have I been a bad parent? And of course, worrying is at its worst in the middle of the night.

Situations involving alcohol, drugs, or cigarettes can be some of the "hottest" to handle, and the most in need of a calm approach. When a "hot" predicament with a teen is multiplied by the stirred-up emotions of the parents, the result can be unwise, knee-jerk parental reactions. While there are no ideal solutions for dicey dilemmas with teens, here are ideas to try for dealing with some common predicaments.

A laid-back dad lets kids drink at his apartment. There's one in almost every group: The parent who believes that teens will be teens and that they're going to drink anyway. In a "pick your poison" decision, he concludes that it's safer for them to knock back a few in the home, in which case there's no driving involved and there's some degree of oversight. Other parents aren't quite as overt, but likewise assume that since drinking is inevitable, they'll simply turn a blind eye to what's going on in the rec room. In a nanosecond, teens figure out where the fun or lax house is and know just where to head to drink. And where there's drink, there is usually smoke — of all flavors.

This approach poses a real quandary for parents. Let's say that a disapproving mom has gotten wind that her former spouse is letting their 16-year-old daughter drink in his apartment with friends. Mom's temptation might be to launch into Dad, telling him in so many words that it's illegal; he's trying to be the fun guy; it's thoughtless, selfish, immature parenting; all the other parents are talking about him; and he needs to be thinking more about their daughter and her health. These are the sort of loaded remarks you might say to an ex and would probably want to say to another parent, but wouldn't have the gumption.

A Calm Approach: Even if you and your ex are apples and oranges on this issue, try to figure out a way to be on the same parenting team. Approach it respectfully, which is less likely to put him on the defensive. (The same would be true for another parent, of course.)

Stay in a questioning mode about potential problems with comments like "I know you care about our daughter and you realize that if drinking gets started early, it can get worse, so have you thought about where this could go?" "What policies will you have so that the drinking won't get out of hand?" "How do you feel about the liability if someone gets hurt?" Remind Dad that if his becomes the "party house," every kid who wants to drink could show up, and with cell phones, a party can ramp up and get out of control. The point is not to chasten, but to get him thinking about the big downsides to this permissive approach.

Although being nice may feel like saccharine in your mouth, this approach may prove effective. And chances are that natural consequences—like a big beer stain on his good couch or a stolen wallet—may eventually curb his indulgent behavior.

Parents leave town trusting that all will be well. Many parents believe that if they hire a responsible college student or young former nanny to hold down the fort with their teen while they're away, everything will be business as usual. Or, parents may let their teen stay with another teen's family, locking up their own home and assuming their child would never, ever sneak into the home. If all has gone well in the past and their teen isn't a high-energy, "out there" social kid, parents can be lulled into complacency.

Might you be in this group? Even if your teen doesn't instigate the merrymaking, word gets out (those cell phones!): "Lizzie's parents are out of town!" Teens are on the lookout for a place to have a party involving substance use.

A Calm Approach: First of all, hire a sharp, no-nonsense older woman as a sitter, since most college kids don't have it in them to be a bear about "no parties." Your teen may be as pure as the driven snow, but it's still risky to allow her to stay at a friend's house and leave your home empty without some kind of additional oversight. An empty house is an invitation for teens to figure out how to goose the system, breaking into their own house to have "just a few friends over" while Mom and Dad are away.

Should you leave town, let your teen know in the friendliest way possible that you are going to put out an all-points alert to friends and neighbors to watch the house. Batten down the hatches. Have multiple backups and eyes on your teen and the house, and arrange for drive-bys to check for funny business. Fair warning!

A 15-year-old teen wants her parent's permission to attend a party with alcohol. Let's say you're the parent of a ninth-grader, a good kid who has always been up front with you. As a freshman, she was ecstatic to make the varsity basketball team and, subsequently, to be invited to the post-season celebration. She admits, "I want to go. I know there will be drinking, but I can handle it. If you say 'no' to these things, I'm going to start needing to lie to you."

A parent's natural inclination is to be impressed with the teen's candor and forthright approach. Wanting to preserve honesty and open communication in the relationship, you might go along with this dubious proposal, trusting her to abstain and be safe, but should you?

A Calm Approach: Teens routinely put their parents in this kind of pinch, especially good kids who want to do something risky or illegal with a clean conscience. It gets them off the hook for taking personal responsibility because, after all, they have Mom's or Dad's consent.

Remember that no matter how convincing their plea, ninth-graders are young and inexperienced, and despite their best intentions, they don't always know what they're getting into. These are tough calls when it's a family's first kid in high school, since parents also lack experience and may make a decision that is naïve in retrospect.

While it's true that some exposure to the drunken-party scene—teens slobbering and throwing up on themselves—can be a big eye opener and turn-off, most teens will run into this on their own, hardly needing a parent's go-ahead to gain this experience.

In the end, some parenting situations are simply a loss; you'll have to be in the doghouse with your kid. Try saying something like "There may come a time when I believe you have the skills up and running to handle this kind of situation, but you're in ninth grade, and these kids are mostly juniors and seniors. I'm saying 'no.' It's your choice to lie, but I'll take action if I discover it. I have to stick to my guns on what I believe to be in your best interest. I know it's rough and that this is an important party and a huge deal. I will have to live with the fact that you're going to be pretty mad at me about this."

A mom is worried sick about her son's drug use. A son's email is open, and Mom sees a message referring to his sale of a bag of weed to another teen. Not only have the son's grades been down, he has been moody, sleeping a lot, and highly uncommunicative. Previously, he was caught with weed and a bong in his gym bag. Dad has become tongue-tied because he doesn't want to add to the fighting. When Mom tries to talk to her son about the email, asking if he's selling, he throws her off, making a lame excuse and wheedling his way out of it, the same way he did with the bong and the found stash. Mom persists, telling her son how worried she is about him. He says weed is better than alcohol, and they head into another argument. Afraid of losing her relationship with her son, Mom tries to keep talking, but it never goes well.

A Calm Approach: Families can become used to a rocky situation, acclimating over time to the slowly declining grades and terrible attitude, not realizing how bad things really are. When at all in doubt, seek a professional evaluation. Don't try yet another conversation about drug use, because a dependent teen will deny it, and around you'll go.

Behaviors associated with drug abuse include academic or school behavior problems; disruptive behaviors; changes of friendships to socialize with peers suspected of substance use; unusual secretiveness or irresponsible behaviors; loss of interest in previous extracurricular activities; leaving telltale evidence. What's confusing is that these behaviors don't automatically mean that a teen should go to rehab, because they could also indicate family problems, depression, or other disorders. Only an evaluation by a professional specializing in this area can sort out what it all means.

A 10th-grader comes home drunk for the first time. We should know that it's coming, since experimenting with substances is "normal" for teens, yet few parents feel prepared when their teen staggers into the house, slurring words and reeking of stale beer. There's a sense of urgency to get all the answers on the spot: "Where did you get it?" "Who were you with?" "How much did you drink?" "Who was driving?" Riled up in the heat of the moment, some parents make quick work of stating a punishment: "You're grounded!"

A Calm Approach: No one should try to have a rational conversation with an inebriated kid. If needed, put him in the shower, make sure he's not going to get sick, and then let him sleep. This approach will buy you time to sort out possible consequences and plan your moves for putting him in the hot seat.

When the next day comes, as with all loaded times with teens, stay fairly quiet and hear what the teen has to say first. Be the dispassionate judge and clue them in ahead of time, letting them know that the severity of the punishment will depend on their degree of self-reflection and willingness to assume responsibility for mistakes. Remorseful teens can sometimes be harder on themselves than parents might be. Typically, teens are grounded, and skillful parents can sometimes turn restricted time into a chance to do something enjoyable together. And if parents see fit to give time off for good behavior, it can sweeten the relationship.

Although it doesn't work as well when teens and parents have a rocky relationship, this approach makes it more likely that the teen will engage in the right spirit with a less defensive and minimizing attitude. Once the teen is in the hot seat, if he thinks getting drunk is no big deal, you'll have to show him it is with larger consequences. But if he is wise, self-critical, and contrite, and can speak with conviction about how he's going to avoid these situations in the future, you can be more merciful.

A high school senior seems to be able to handle some weekend drinking. Parents realize that their senior, who otherwise has his life together, uses alcohol recreationally, drinking with friends on occasion at parties. When questioned about this habit, he claims emphatically that they use designated drivers, that everything stays under control, and that it's no more harmful than his parents' cocktail hour. Despite their disapproval, the parents can't identify any obvious negative consequences associated with his drinking, since he's making good grades, keeping up with extracurricular activities, and doesn't miss curfew.

As unsettled as the parents are, they feel that there isn't anything they can do or say. Their son is 18, headed to college next year, and they can't keep him home every Saturday night.

A Calm Approach: With a younger teen, parents can justifiably crack down on substances, since no one knows where its use might lead, and concerns that it could progress are very valid. Although parents should never be at ease with any teen drinking, it's trickier with an older teen who has a track record for using alcohol moderately and responsibly. Plus, even though many of today's teens are conscientious about using designated drivers, it's not the airtight system they lead parents to believe.

Rather than doing nothing, keep the conversations going. Try a relational approach that implies "I'm doing this for you, now you do this for me." Have talks that go something like this: "You're comfortable with your drinking, but I'm not. Still, I always feel more comfortable if I'm more in the loop with what's up with your social life. Let's do a swap. I am trusting you to be a good decision maker and in exchange, you can be talking to me more about what's going on. You don't need to name names, but I'd like you to tell me how you're handling various situations to reassure me that you are showing good judgment."

Proceed to ask questions that will both stimulate thinking and provide a sliver of assurance. "How do you handle it at parties when you think police could come?" "What would the implication of an MIP ("minor in possession" citation) on your record be for your future?" "What do you and your friends do when someone is drinking too much?"

Parents can still be stern with relatively mature older teens. "I'm not going to keep you home at 18, but I don't want you to think I'm taking this lightly.

Alcohol affects the growing brain. I'm going to be watching those curfews, kissing you good night, and I reserve the right to withdraw privileges if I think things are getting out of hand."

A parent catches her sixth-grader with a cigarette. What middle-schooler hasn't tried a cigarette? So common is this experience—for every teen in every generation—that a mom who discovers that her daughter has taken her first puff may go easy on her. She might admit to her daughter that she remembers going down to the ravine and trying a cigarette herself. As the situation amicably plays out, the daughter says, "Don't worry, Mom, I won't do it again." Mom understands and lets it ride, assuming this will be an isolated episode.

A Calm Approach: Taking a fierce approach with a high-schooler is dicey, because they're capable of responding adamantly and confidently that they can handle the risk. With your average sixth-grader, if you're not routinely on her back, it's all right every now and then to throw the book at her, especially knowing what we do about nicotine addiction and teens.

Consider an assertive approach: "I cannot take this lightly. This is huge. Do you know your brain is different after one cigarette? Every cigarette gives way a little bit to your wanting another." Remind her that the tobacco industry is going after teens to get them hooked. Pull out some statistics on the health hazards of smoking. To raise her awareness, insist that she review ads with you to scrutinize how they try to convince teens that smoking makes them look sexy and cool.

Your teen wants to know whether you inhaled. Here's a tight spot that comes up like clockwork: You're hanging out with your teen in the kitchen in a friendly way, and he pops the question, "Did you drink as a teen?" Parents can feel at a loss about how much to tell, and in the spirit of openness, you might go ahead and admit to sowing a few wild oats. How prudent is this?

A Calm Approach: In truth, there's no easy "yes" or "no." A general guideline, however, is that if your teen is just fishing for information, there are advantages to staying circumspect and keeping your experiences to yourself. It doesn't matter whether you never touched drugs in your life or you smoked pot like a chimney during college; the question is whether your teen stands to benefit from your disclosure. Because adolescents are more likely to learn from their own smart moves, stupid moves, and trial-and-error moves, it's naive for us to think that revealing our pasts might actually protect our kids from making the same dumb mistakes we made. Often, it's downright distracting.

Hold off on describing your own indiscretions until you can make an argument in your head that there will be some real gain. When a teen is in trouble or experiencing a crisis and is overwhelmed with shame and remorse, a disclosure about your own fall from grace can be an incredible gift. Be specific about how you suffered and what you learned. To simply say, "I've made mistakes" is a throw-away line. Admitting to similar mistakes is all the more helpful to a traumatized kid if it comes from a parent who doesn't share war stories.

Write a Caring Note to Your Teen

At some point, almost all teens will be staring at a vape, a drink, a pill, or some other drug, deciding whether or not to give it a try. Instead of whistling in the dark hoping for the best, parents can meet this prospect head on by writing a note to their teen.

The example that follows can be used as a crib sheet for parents to compose their own letter to their teens. This letter hits a number of important points, among them that the parent has a strong preference against substance use; is realistic about the possibilities of the teen's use of substances; cares most of all about their teen's health and safety; can be called any time; asks them to think hard, because the harm is real, and life can turn on a dime in a moment of bad judgment. A letter like this one creates a bridge between "please don't" and "but if you do."

Dear (Son or Daughter),

As you enter your teen years, you'll be faced with decisions about drinking and using drugs. If it were my choice, I'd choose that you do neither, but I realize you'll be in situations where you'll be choosing for yourself.

I'll skip the extreme statements and scary exaggerations, because I know that many teens try substances and that having a couple of drinks won't necessarily lead to drug abuse. But it still worries me, and I don't take even a little experimentation lightly. Mainly, I want to emphasize being smart about your health and safety.

You'll hear a lot about the dangers of drugs like cocaine and heroin. Because alcohol and cigarettes are more commonly used, there's a false sense that they're not dangerous. But they are the substances most likely to take lives in the long run, and the earlier people start to use either, especially as teens, the greater the possibility that their health will be harmed.

With even one cigarette, there could be a tiny change in your brain chemistry that will make you want another, and then another later on. Most smokers want to stop, and they wish they could turn back the clock and never have started. You still have a chance not to start. Think about even a little bit of smoking very, very carefully.

My message about marijuana, alcohol, and other substances is similar. Think very carefully before you try them. It might seem like it's going to be fun or interesting, but it doesn't necessarily turn out that way. Marijuana can make people incredibly self-conscious or paranoid. You know how dangerous driving under the influence of drugs is, because substances affect the way people think and behave. They end up taking risks—with driving, illegal activity, and sex—that they would have never otherwise considered. It's so scary how good people can be scarred for life in the blink of an eye because of something they did when their judgment was impaired by alcohol or drugs.

Please trust me when I say that I want you to talk to me about any of your concerns. I'll pick you up anytime from any situation that makes you uncomfortable, no questions asked.

These days, downing shots of alcohol and playing drinking games have become common, but I want you to consider not participating. Ultimately, if you decide to drink, moderation is extremely important, since drinking more than two or three drinks is considered a binge and that's where really impaired judgment and trouble set in.

Reflecting on all of your decisions—before you're in a place where drinking, partying, and sexual activity are happening—is critical. You're smart enough to have noticed that when socializing revs up, people make impulsive choices they may later regret. I don't expect you to be perfect, but I do hope you're putting a lot of thought into your life choices, especially the ones that have to do with health and safety.

Love,
(Mom or Dad)

Actions That Speak Louder than Words

There's no single message and no single parenting move that will completely eliminate the possibility that a teen might make a bad decision in an arousing situation. To reduce harm, parents need to approach teen substance use from many different angles. In addition to a parent's ever watchful eye, the following attitudes and actions can make a difference.

Make the connections happen. There is magic in connections. All the research in this area of study shows that a warm, cohesive, and caring parent-child relationship can protect kids practically across the board, particularly with negative risk taking. A strong and caring parent-teen relationship, where parents monitor their children and establish effective limits, is associated with fewer teen pregnancies, less school failure, and fewer emotional difficulties (depression and anxiety, for example).

Be confident that a few good rules, consistently maintained, will go a long way. Family rules and policies can be tailored to your teen and her track record. If you know you have a wild one, keep those fence posts tight. Stay up to speed on your teen's comings and goings and get cell numbers for friends and their parents for tracking your teen's whereabouts. Do an occasional spot check. Enforce curfews and ask your teen to give you a peck on the cheek upon returning home so you can get a whiff of his breath. "Monitoring" is the magic word used in the research to describe the families who manage to keep their kids on the safe(r) side of the risk-taking continuum.

Watch your own p's and q's (pints and quarts). Teens observe a parent's intake like a hawk. They know if Dad has had a glass of wine before getting behind the wheel. Our words mean nothing if we're contradicting them with our actions. It may seem extreme, but smart parents lock up any alcohol in the house, because teens will often pilfer. To limit exposure, don't ask teens to serve alcohol to adults at parties.

Keep an eye on your teen's friends. Know whom your teen is with, where they're going, and what they intend to do together. Keep a record of friends' contact information and touch base with their parents now and then. If your teen's friends are using substances, your teen probably is, too. If you have evidence that substance use occurs with certain friends, restricting contact with them is legitimate.

Reach out to the village. Rely on the parental grapevine for all it's worth, and also stay connected to your broader community. With the realities of teen development and teen risk taking, it's almost impossible for parents to protect their sons and daughters on their own around the clock. We're our kids' primary keepers, but the second line of defense is their community of caring and watchful adults—from the neighbor who alerts us to some funny business, to the teacher who mentors on responsibility, to a best friend's mother who still thinks a teen is the cat's pajamas, even if he's blown it big time and publicly.

Not too many years ago, when Mrs. Smith saw Mrs. Johnson's son speeding down the street, she'd call up that mom straight away. Research shows the advantages of bringing these days back. Having gone too far in the opposite direction, we need to be minding each other's business a little bit more. Social organization (as it's called) helps explain why some very disadvantaged neighborhoods can still keep their rates of delinquency relatively low.[5]

Our teens live out in the world, and they're being enticed left and right by more harmful influences and alluring images than we might ever imagine. We do our best as parents to raise kids who are healthy and strong enough to resist, but what teen wouldn't benefit from a little extra protective insulation from a caring community?

We now have a scientific basis for understanding that teens, by their very nature, will take risks and that their brain development process makes such actions particularly rewarding and thrilling. Despite what we know, we still can't keep them under wraps every night, and all the drug education in the world won't be enough to prevent substance use entirely.

The responsibility falls on parents' shoulders to be both vigilant and realistic. In the long run, kids realize that having parents who are "a little strict" is a good thing, as long as you have the positive relationship to go with it. When you catch your teen drinking or smoking, stay calm and rein them in. Teens sometimes know subconsciously when they need to be pulled back; they can send out signals for us to slow them down, such as when they leave evidence, act in ways that make being caught likely, or make insane requests they don't actually expect us to grant.

Parents walk a fine line between accepting teens as they stumble through experimenting with substances and showing strong disapproval and imposing limits and consequences as needed. In other words, we're not one of those parents who goes berserk with the discovery of their teen's substance use or one who shrugs it off with a "Kids will drink." Parents who do the hard work of striking that balance can make all the difference.

CHAPTER 14

When Everyone Is Completely Stressed Out

It's the witching hour in the family kitchen with a busy evening ahead, but Gina, a mother of three, has taken extra measures to make everything come together. Setting aside some important emails until after dinner, Gina dashed home early from work, drove a carpool for her older son, and is now preparing dinner for everyone to eat in a flash before her husband heads out to a mandatory soccer meeting.

The phone rings. It's another mom. She's terribly sorry—knows it's last minute—but she has to take her elderly mother to the hospital, so could Gina please pick up their daughters? Gina is searching for her keys when her younger son comes into the room, awash in tears. A report is due tomorrow, and he spilled juice on his laptop, crashing his system. He has lost all his work and is hysterical about starting over.

The phone rings again. "Your dog has jumped the fence and is out in the street," a neighbor reports. The kicker comes when Gina's husband calls, apologizing profusely, to say that he was pulled aside by a coworker on his way out the door, left work way later than planned, and is stuck in horrendous traffic and won't be home in time for the soccer meeting. Parental attendance is required for their son to qualify for the team, so . . .

Sound familiar?

Stressed, if not overwhelmed by hurry-up lifestyles, many parents feel pulled in too many directions at once, trying to keep pace with a multitude of schedules, responsibilities, and obligations screaming for attention. If it's not the team fundraiser, it's the son who suddenly needs glasses, or the email from the teacher urgently requesting a conference. Even without kids' agendas, parents have their own gargantuan "to do" lists. Personal time to exercise or just relax would be a dream come true.

Parents can also be dumbfounded by the smorgasbord of options for kids' activities and enrichment—from scouting to water polo to Mandarin Chinese lessons. Our heads spin with the vast abundance of choices, adding to the confusion, stress, and exhaustion. This phenomenon trickles down to mundane areas of life, such as the grocery aisles with their myriad selections. "Should I buy the salsa in the refrigerator section, the one in the health-food section, the one on the shelf with the Mexican food, or the one featured in the display with the chips—and why am I spending time on this?" one wonders. Fewer choices would make life a lot easier.

The ultimate commodity in the 21st century is time. No one seems to have enough of this precious resource. Families with teens are in a particular fix because it takes extra time to create some positive moments to compensate for all the negative ones that come with the territory of parenting teens. The developmental business of adolescence—the complaining, resisting, rudeness, and noncompliance—eats away at efforts to have good times together. As it turns out, "quality" time often happens serendipitously, but only out of a large quantity of time.

Relationships take time, period. A frenetic lifestyle compromises all the goals and recommendations in this book. To negotiate the minefields described in each chapter, our minds need to be calm so that we can solve problems astutely. Riled up by an incident, an attitude, or some infuriating experience, we're not biologically programmed to cool off and regulate our emotions in a split second. Most of the stupid moves we make as parents and later regret spring from moments when our buttons are pushed, our adrenaline is rushing, our brains are flooding, and we neglect to zip our lips. We need to take a break, remove ourselves from the heat of the moment, practice the CALM technique (Cool down; Assess options; Listen with empathy; Make a plan), and slow our heart rates down. Only then can we choose our approach wisely and show empathy and understanding for our loved ones.

Ask most parents what they value most in life and they'll answer, "My family," yet we don't always walk this talk. When friends ask, "How are you?" few parents respond in a way that says, "I'm living my family values and spending lots of quality time with my loved ones in healthful ways." Most describe how busy they are with work, home upkeep, crazy kid schedules, commutes, or carpools.

How can parents that are struggling with a time famine figure out how to use their time for what is truly best for their family, their children, and themselves? Some moms and dads don't have a moment to take stock, but even when parents do pause to question their harried lifestyle, the story below shows that there's no easy solution.

Family Story: **A Scheduling Dilemma**

Although most parents start off with the idea of raising a "well-rounded" child who participates in different activities, by middle school the pressure is on for full-year training in a single sport. What's a parent to do if a child is supertalented in two sports? And what if she might also want to be in the school band? As hard as it is on their developing bodies, young athletes who want to "succeed" are advised to specialize.

Case in point is 12-year-old Cullen, who thrives on swimming and is up eagerly at the crack of dawn most mornings for his workout. As if that weren't enough, his parents now have to decide whether he should advance to the next level, despite the toll it would take on their family and potentially on him. Neither maniacal nor unusual, here is your average family with active, healthy kids, deliberating the pros and cons of upping the athletic ante. Do these parents just say "no" to their son's pursuit of excellence for the sake of family sanity?

Dad: You won't believe this. Cullen's swim coach has invited him to join the elite squad. He'd be the youngest one on the team! Coach Mac said his butterfly stroke could be developed to make him an Olympic-level competitor.

Mom: Mac has hinted the same to me, but Cullen is only in sixth grade! He's already up every morning at 5:30 to get to the 6:15 workout, and this would mean adding three evenings a week. This sounds crazy to me.

Dad: Yes, but swimming is all he can talk about. How can we stand in the way of his talent? With all the trouble that teens get into these days, we should be glad that he wants to be in the pool and has this healthy outlet.

Mom: I think about the same things. On the one hand, I'm proud and want to support Cullen all the way. Mac's comment about Cullen's perfect stroke really excites me. On the other, I'm second-guessing our lifestyle all the time. I never thought I'd be one of those moms who practically lives in the car with her kids. Amanda loves her gymnastics, and Cullen loves his swim team, but they're both always on the move and always tired. I'll feel guilty either way we go on this decision. We'll either be down to eating one meal together a week on Sundays, if that, or depriving our son of his chance for the Olympics.

Dad: I know. We're already too busy, and I can't imagine how we'd work out the carpooling. I suppose Cullen could get a ride with the earlier workout bunch that leaves from school and pack a dinner.

Mom: He already "packs" breakfast and lunch—he'll forget what a warm dinner is! Because of everyone's schedules, if Cullen does this, he'll spend nearly every night of the week either working out or being in the car while one of us takes Amanda to her club. Amanda's not that great at gymnastics, but she deserves just as much of our energy as Cullen. She already complains that the "pool rules" and takes jabs at me for training the "great one." All of his trophies have taken a toll on her self-esteem.

Dad: I see that, too, and that's why I keep doing the Girl Y Guides, even though it monopolizes so many weekends. The thing that nags at me is that if we say "no" to Cullen, I fear that at age 20, he'll look back and feel like we took an opportunity of a lifetime away from him.

Mom: Yeah, either that or feel like swimming robbed him of his childhood. Remember when we swore that we'd go out together as a couple every week, always have family dinners, and spend lots of downtime with our kids? How did we get on this treadmill?

What could be better than parents helping their children find their passions, develop their gifts, and build the skills that enhance selfhood, self-esteem, and future opportunities? As great as all that sounds, it can put enormous pressure on everyone.

How do parents decide what to add or subtract from the family schedule? When do we let our kids cram more into an already packed schedule? When do we allow them to quit an activity that could be advantageous to them down the road? When do we insist that they persevere through a rough schedule? When do we encourage them to drop an activity so they can try out something potentially more promising? Parents toil over such questions, especially during the teen years when the stakes seem higher. Since no one has a crystal ball, these quandaries can lead to obsessions, power struggles, and analysis paralysis. Even if 51 percent of our brain makes one decision, the other 49 percent is agonizing about the direction not chosen.

Many decisions have a big sting either way. Cullen's parents, for example, must choose between adding stress and hardship to their lives or shutting the door on an opportunity that might change the course of their son's life. And when heady things like the Olympics are part of the equation, the values related to a calmer home life are easily lost in the shuffle.

How can families settle on a direction? Try to get the big picture by reflecting on the following questions:

- Do you see any symptoms that suggest a problem? A compulsion to stay with workouts in spite of injuries and doctors' recommendations? Frequent meltdowns? Increasing illness? Constant fatigue?
- Is your teen missing significant experiences that will create big holes in his development? Is there a lack of friendships? Inadequate investment in academics? No time for investing in other values, like religion, time in nature, or service?

- What's the mood of the family? Is stress getting to everyone? Are family members at each other's throats? Lots more arguing?
- Who is behind the push? Primarily the teen? You, the parent? Or a coach/mentor?
- How "emotional" is this decision? Could something be blindsiding you? Is your own ego too wrapped up in this?

Assess all the reasons, pro and con, to see how they stack up. If things lean in the negative direction, then consider giving something a rest. Your teen may be talented and may want to forge ahead, but it's still fine to pull back if it's not a prudent decision for your family. Though teens may balk, at some point, we have to assume they'll be able to adapt. Try saying something reassuring like "We're disappointed, too, but we're confident you can handle it."

On the plus side, if circumstances are tolerable despite the craziness and there's enough of a buffer to the stress that a ramped-up schedule will impose on the family, it may be worth the stretch. Still, go forward with some awareness of your motives, which may include the reasons below.

Why We Put Up With the Rat Race

Why not just cut back, cancel some activities, ease the pressure, and kick back a little? For all of our complaints and misery, we have reasons, some better than others, for keeping up the hectic pace and ramped-up lifestyles.

Families can benefit from taking a hard look at what is driving their pace. What are the supposed gains for all your pains? Are you getting enough out of it? Are the reasons good enough to justify the downsides?

A lot of complex reasons lie behind the harried lifestyles of many families. Here are some of the most common:

Dreams of future opportunities for our children. Compared to our own moms and dads, we're a much more child-focused generation of parents, concerned about academic achievement, talent development, and skill building. Some parents stay in the fast lane, showering their kids with enriching opportunities and advantages because they believe that somehow, something good will come of it. Many parents believe their teens need a special edge (a sport, talent, or credential) to be accepted into a "good" college. Because most parents want the best for their kids and will do whatever is within their reach, deciding where to stop is no easy matter.

The rush. Some people love the jolt of adrenaline that comes from over-extending and overreaching more than others. Without question, it can be gratifying to nail a challenging array of demands, from working to volunteering, to managing the kids and the house, to knocking items off the to-do list. While some recoil from the rush and admirably pull the plug, others are revved up by it and make parenting into a competitive sport, organizing zillions of activities on a spreadsheet schedule. By nature, humans are competitive, and the thrills of achievement and accomplishment can be one of the highest highs out there. Nevertheless, much has been written about the harms of overparenting and overscheduling kids. Yet we still do it because our kids can be reflections of ourselves, and fueling them fuels us.

The dirty little secret: Family time isn't always wonderful and rewarding. What is it that keeps us preoccupied with things other than the family? Could there be something we're avoiding? Many parents claim they're too busy to cook, but if truth be told, family dinners aren't always full of joy. By skipping family meals, you don't have to contend with a grumpy kid who may be rude at the table and complain about the food, and then argue until he's blue in the face about cleaning up. As difficult as it is to admit, online poker, emailing, or clicking through the TV options can be more stimulating than family time; plus, these diversions allow us to hide from the adversities of family life. When everyone in the family is in the same flow, happy and content, it's the best thing on earth, but a lot of the time, we're out of sync with our teens. The best we can do while prioritizing this mixed bag is to remember that, no matter what, time together still matters.

Pure anxiety. Anxiety comes from many sources: from doing something, from not doing something, and from indecision over which way to go. Parents wonder about the secret sauce that will make their kid successful. Sometimes we maintain a questionable status quo because change itself creates anxiety. Parents fret about what their family might miss out on if they leave an unsatisfying yet lucrative job or take a pay cut to spend more time with the kids. "How will we pay the bills?" "Will we have to move into a different neighborhood with more crime, lower-quality schools, and negative peer influence?" "If I cut back, am I cheating my child in some way?" "Am I lazy or selfish if I don't want to add scouts or summer science school to the schedule?"

Feeling like a better parent because of sacrifices. Parents endure all kinds of hardships in order to provide more and better opportunities for their kids. We suffer the pangs of a stressful lifestyle because it's what good parents do, putting up with the commute to live in the suburbs with a better school system, paying for classes and new goodies for the children, and sacrificing time for one's self. Rest and relaxation (and sex) are way down on the list.

Following the crowd. Social beings that we are, part of our "human nature" is to be influenced by what others are doing, whether that means getting the TV with the newest technology or moving to a bigger house. Conformity has been studied in a variety of behaviors, such as jay-walking, teen linguistics, and shopping patterns, and the conclusion is the same: People are mimics, taking cues from others. For the most part, this is a good thing, because it leads us to follow rules and incorporate new inventions and ways of thinking into our lives (technology, values on human rights, environmental conservation). But the downside is that instead of choosing lifestyles deliberately, we plod along under group influence. Even, for example, if our personal values tell us to put on the brakes, nurture our marriages, and raise our children in wholesome ways, it's tough to gear down when everyone else is gearing up.

The slow creep. No matter how hyped up, once a hectic lifestyle takes root, it becomes the new norm, and we lose a sense of how crazy things may have become. Consider everything that we've piled on, little by little, over the last generation: entertainment centers, cell phones for each child, multiple cars in one family, a constantly updated wardrobe. This is a lot to keep up. Various circumstances play into the slow creep. Although technology has made us more efficient, screen activities consume more than their fair share of time, leaving us less face-to-face time with friends and family. We're less comfortable with the idea of boredom, leaving very little time unscheduled to see what might develop. Sophisticated advertising triggers our inner materialist, urging us toward greater heights as consumers. One analogy for our lifestyle is the "frog in the cooking pot." Up goes the temperature, little by little, so gradually that the frog gets used to it and doesn't jump out while he can. Ultimately, conditions are so hot and he's so weakened that it's too late for him to leap to his own rescue.

Without question, we all need to stay engaged in life, using our talents, supporting our kids in their activities, and contributing to our communities. Overscheduling is a problem, but so is underscheduling. Let's hear it for activities for teens! Given their high spirits and risk-taking potential, teens need ways to harness their energy and use their time in positive ways. It's only a problem when we've gone too far in one direction.

Flourishing lives are a matter of balance. Some busyness is a good thing, for teens and parents alike, but more isn't necessarily better. What does it take to slow it all down?

Crafting a Calmer Home

Maria has totaled the car, and it was her fault. Driving several middle-schoolers to dress rehearsal for the school play and running late, she was heedlessly tailgating, and when the car in front of her stopped abruptly, she swerved to avoid a collision, careening off the road. Thank goodness no one was hurt, but to add insult to injury, Maria was given a ticket for reckless driving.

Shaken up by the wreck, she had to deal not only with her own and the children's fright, but with other kids' parents, who were as upset with her as she was with herself. She had endangered everyone's lives.

This crisis sets Maria to mulling over her behavior for the last six months. Running an inventory, she thinks about how she recently screamed at the top of her lungs at a guy who nabbed her parking place. He was a jerk, but it was uncharacteristic of her to become unglued over a thing like this.

Day in and day out, she's also been yelling at the kids. Her mild-mannered ways have given way to constant irritation with the smallest thing. When the kids fail to pitch in or do things they are asked to do, she no longer has it in herself to come up with a solution, resorting instead to nagging and getting madder.

She loves her husband, but is feeling a lot of resentment toward him, not always warranted. Steamed up, she makes little predictions in her head such as "I'll bet he didn't unload the dishwasher" or "He probably just threw his dirty clothes on the floor," only to discover otherwise. Maria sees that she has been looking for a place to dump her grievances, jumping all over him when things go wrong.

Sleep is another thing. Never getting more than six hours of sleep, she feels strung out and exhausted most of the time. And she is furious with herself because she is months behind in her thank-you notes and remiss in calling her friends back.

Her mind stirs with thoughts of how neglectful she is as a parent, not finding time to talk to her kids about important matters. Clearly, her son is ignoring some of the parameters they have established for his online use, but instead of following through and enforcing consequences, she just continues to nag. Maria suspects that her daughter isn't being truthful with her whereabouts. Something is off, and it probably pertains to her daughter's new crush, but she can't find a minute to sniff it out.

Maria has received a ticket for reckless driving, but she feels so out of control that she may as well have been cited for reckless living. That, in a nutshell, typifies what family life has become for many. Families are dealing with more than full plates, making due, coping with exhaustion, and catching their breath in lulls between storms.

Typically, it takes a crisis like Maria's or a last straw before we realize we're out of control and need a new plan. But even if you haven't yet arrived at that point, why not call a time-out for reflection to see whether you're running your life or life is running you? Could you be nearing a point where things could catch up and take a toll—if not a car wreck, then some kind of life wreck?

Although a whole new plan may be unrealistic and unnecessary, many families could benefit from some adjusting to calm the pace, even with a move as minimal as declaring email off limits on Sundays. The idea isn't to go from all to nothing, sitting around the house in idleness, but rather to shift from too much of everything to everything in moderation. Parents need to keep their kids involved in sports and other activities, stay active in their community, and maintain their own interests. But before adding one more thing, consider subtracting something at the same time. Ideally, we should be deliberate about choosing how we use our time with the goal of family health.

What does cutting back involve? The pointers below can apply to a variety of pull-back situations, like when families need to tighten their financial belt. Changing course will include:

An act of will. Any change requires insight into what it will involve, recognizing that it will be hard. For everything you stand to gain, you'll also lose out, and you may feel threatened and anxious about things you're not doing, like the party you skip because it's family night, the item you don't buy because you're not working extra hours, or the letdown you feel because you're no longer the top volunteer in the spotlight. Because of everything you'll miss, you may need to reward yourself now and then with the thought "I get to have a calm home and enjoy my family." By concentrating on your kids and family like they're your most valued customer, you'll be living this value.

Organization and creativity. A calmer life doesn't happen without clear decisions around the give and take of what you can and can't do. You might, for example, decide to live with a messier house or more weeds in the garden so that you can go to exercise class. Or, you may determine to reduce stress by staying within your budget, even though this means that the kids wear hand-me-down sports uniforms instead of new ones.

Organizing, itself, takes time. You'll need to hold weekly family business meetings for synchronizing everyone's schedules and calendars, assigning household duties, reviewing family policies and choices, and evaluating how things are going. Consider time management strategies, such as allowing an extra 10 minutes to get out the door instead of cutting it close, screaming at the kids like a maniac, "We're late! Hurry up!"

Realize that unless you unplug in a deliberate way, time will be chewed up by the next thing in front of you. Typically, family time is made up of the leftovers. Instead, create an inviolable block of time dedicated to family time first. You might decide to set aside three nights a week with no activities, and if that conflicts with chess club, then no chess club. Or you could dedicate one part of a weekend for a family outing of some sort. And in a two-parent family, couples need to clear the schedule for a weekly date.

More responsibility for the kids. Overprotectiveness has mushroomed during the last generation or two. With fears of "stranger danger," parents are inclined to keep the kids inside (with screens) instead of sending them out on their own. Many moms and dads feel like chauffeurs, delivering kids door to door, wary of having them take the bus or ride their bikes. Making kids run an errand means letting them loose in the big, bad world. Some parents don't want to burden their children with responsibilities because it would rob them of enrichment opportunities.

But what if the kids chipped in more with the idea that many hands make light work, as the saying goes? Perhaps the kids could be given dinner duty for one meal a week. And, on the night they cook, they get to invite a friend over.

Overprotectiveness can make for fragile kids who are less resilient. Resilience is a child's capacity to cope with adversity, negotiate challenges, and achieve well-being, not necessarily in spite of life's stressors but sometimes because of them. Many parents desire to bubble-wrap their children, leaving them devoid of the opportunity to develop this highly desirable ability. Challenges—and some level of stress—build talents, skills, and hardiness. As important as family nurturing and a calm home are, so is the chance to surmount hurdles and develop coping skills for the natural adversities of life.

Wising up to the impact of stress. In any fast-paced life, the body takes a hit from stress through a cascading series of neurochemicals, with short-term and long-term effects. Extra-stress cortisol and adrenaline are released from our adrenal glands whenever we feel a sense of urgency, whether it's from having too much to do or worrying about the kids. Physiologically, our heart and breathing rates increase, blood pressure rises, muscles become tense, and we're poised to take action, sometimes in ways that bail us out—like running to the meeting so we're not late—and sometimes in very unbecoming ways—like being rude at the post office because of the long line.

Being on alert is advantageous when dealing with threats that require this boost or "charge" of hormones, and it served our ancestors well when they needed to pounce and save babies from cougars. But this system, deep in our DNA, is far from ideal for coping with the constant, low-level annoyances in our daily lives. After years of chronic activation, stress responses wear down the body, resulting in symptoms like impaired memory, a weakened immune system, high blood pressure, stomach ulcers, skin problems, digestive problems, and sleep difficulties. Research has documented how the extreme stress of even a few "adverse child events" (known as ACEs) can result in higher rates of lung disease, cancer, heart disease, and diabetes than in groups not suffering that trauma.[1]

Sleep deprivation is a huge problem, affecting mood, concentration, memory, and learning. As detrimental as it is for adults, teens can be in worse straits. During puberty, melatonin, a hormone that regulates circadian rhythms, kicks in about two hours later in the evening compared to childhood. Teens fall asleep later, even though they have to get up early for school.

Stress is like the rotting wood under the garage—you may not be aware of it, but it's eroding the foundation, inevitably undermining individual and family health. What to do? Exercise is one obvious answer, but some highly driven people exercise profusely only to return to being anxious, driven, impatient, and irritable. A movement called "mindfulness" offers some ideas by combining principles of meditation with progressive body relaxation and deep breathing to help people clear their minds of toxic thoughts, slow down enough to be "present," and gain some physiological control of their bodies. With the ubiquitous stress in most people's lives, almost anyone could benefit from these kinds of practices.[2]

A Strategic Plan for Building Family Health

Businesses and organizations devise strategies to improve their performances—doesn't a family deserve as much strategic planning as any job? How do you know whether you're being a "good parent"? Whether you're creating a calm, caring, supportive home? Checklists can provide some specifics to gauge how we're doing.

Below is a plan for family health. Each of the core goals (A through F) is followed by a series of action items that promote the goal. Many parenting manuals contain developmental asset lists, describing behaviors that enhance children's development. Similar in kind, the lists are all based on research. What follows is a synthesis of this information:

ABCs of Family Health

A. Adopt good habits for a larger quantity of time and more quality time with your family.
- Prioritize time with your teen without distractions.
- Limit TV, computer games, and media exposure.
- Model and arrange for reading time.
- Prepare meals and eat dinner together.
- Assign chores at home and serve others in the community together.
- Support mental and physical health by prioritizing exercise, sleep, nutrition, exposure to nature, and self-calming activities.

B. Be a supporter of your teen's scholastic development.
- Be engaged and involved with your teen's school.
- Provide a positive learning environment, which may include a "study hall" policy at home.
- Communicate academic expectations and values.
- If there are school achievement problems, seek consultation.

C. Commit to developing your child's social and emotional competence.
- Supervise teens relative to their ability and track record in handling independence, allowing them to grow and be safe.
- Encourage active involvement in organizations, including teams and clubs in school, volunteering in the community, or participating in a place of worship.
- Know your children's friends and their families.
- Model friendship and social skills.
- Demonstrate gratefulness, respect, and tolerance in everyday life.

D. Develop an authoritative parenting style, which includes warmth in the parent-child relationship, effective communication, and strong parental authority.
- Sustain warmth by showing compassion, empathy, and responsiveness.
- Communicate effectively by validating others' feelings, listening, and

knowing when not to talk.

- Practice techniques to regulate your emotions, including the CALM technique (Cool down; Assess options; Listen with empathy; Make a plan). Avoid talking while "under the influence" of destructive emotions and know that you can choose your words only when not experiencing emotional flooding.
- Avoid intrusiveness and trying to control others' thoughts and feelings.
- Remember the importance of mostly positive interactions, which means picking your battles and maintaining good humor.
- Be thoughtful about how you use parental authority. Maintain structure and supervision; parental unity on policies; appropriate limits and follow-through on consequences; your own moral credibility in areas like alcohol use, conflict resolution, emotional and physical health, and consumer habits.

E. Enhance your family infrastructure.

- Maintain firm emotional boundaries and focus on self-control.
- Avoid favoritism of one child over another, more difficult child.
- Avoid parent-child alliances and siding against another parent/child.
- Focus on accountability to your parenting values, staying firm while under pressure (when, for example, teens plead for more things or indulgences).
- Review family goals and healthful endeavors, and be proactive about adjustments.
- Develop and maintain social support—connections with people and institutions—for everyone in the family.
- Make a calm home a priority.

F. Focus on resilience and the need for lifelong problem solving on delicate issues.

- Be proactive about talking to your teens about sexuality, substance use, violence, and media literacy.
- Know that life always presents problems and that growth results from overcoming adversity, rising to the occasion with compassion, acceptance, and a commitment to relationships.

What keeps families from engaging in an all-encompassing overhaul like this? Time and energy, of course. A crazy lifestyle throws us off course, leaving good intentions and values in the dust. There's also the reality that parenting is extremely hard work, particularly with teens. We may have moments of bliss when it's going well, but it's not always gratifying to be with a cranky teen who is rejecting your positive overtures 90 percent of the time.

Americans are known to chase happiness with the next big thing—the new car, the new kitchen, the fancy outfit. These are things that may make us feel good or look good, but they have very little impact on family health. As it turns out, we have illusions about what we think will make us happy. A number of research studies have established that wealth is not correlated to happiness. An increase in income can initially be a perk, and families certainly need to be able to support themselves and have a cushion, but beyond that level, greater wealth does not generally make people happier or more satisfied. That's because when we have less, we believe that "more" will make us happier, but once we have "more," we habituate to it and then chase the next level of material wealth.

In the end, the best predictor of human happiness involves finding and using our talents and having close and supportive relationships with family and friends. Although simple to say, it takes a lifetime of effort to build and maintain. Develop pastimes together with your teens—sports outings, a favorite show on TV, cooking together—even if it's not exactly how you'd choose to spend your time. Look out over the horizon at the relationship you hope to have with your teens when they're grown and start making it happen now, in spite of all the brattiness and busyness that gets in the way. What do you want your teens to remember about you as a parent? That you were stressed out and hot under the collar, or that you were firm, supportive, and always had their best interest at heart? What values do you want to engender? A craving for things, or characteristics like generosity, self-awareness, and integrity? Above all, think about everything you stand to gain when you slow down and focus on relationships.

Notes

Chapter 1

1. Daniel Offer, *The Psychological World of the Teenager* (New York: Basic Books, 1969). Daniel Offer, E. Ostrov, and K. Howard, *The Adolescent: A Psychological Self-Portrait* (New York: Basic Books, 1981).
2. R.E. Larzelere, A.S. Morris, A.W. Harrist, eds. *Authoritative Parenting: Synthesizing Nurturance and Discipline for Optimal Child Development*. American Psychological Association, 2012.
3. J.M. Resnick, P. Bearman, and R. Blum, et al. "Protecting Adolescents from Harm: Findings from the National Longitudinal Study on Adolescent Health," Journal of the American Medical Association 278 (1997): 823–32.
4. J. Gottman, *The Heart of Parenting: Raising an Emotionally Intelligent Child* (New York: Simon and Schuster, 1997).

Chapter 2

1. Jay Giedd, et al. "Brain Development During Childhood and Adolescence: A Longitudinal MRI Study," Nature Neuroscience 2 (1999): 861–3.
2. D. Yurgelun-Todd, "Inside the Teenage Brain. One Reason Teens Respond Differently to the World: Immature Brain Circuitry." 2003. www.pbs.org/wgbh/pages/frontline/shows/teenbrain/work/onereason
3. R.E. Dahl, "Affect Regulation, Brain Development, and Behavioral/ Emotional Health in Adolescence." CNS Spectrums 6 (1) (2001): 1–12.

Chapter 3

1. J. Allen, C. Moore, G. Kuperminc, and K. Bell, "Attachment and Adolescent Psychosocial Functioning," Child Development 69 (1998): 1406–19. M. Lewis, C. Feiring, and S. Rosenthal, "Attachment over Time," Child Development 71 (2000): 707–20.

Chapter 5

1. www.statisticbrain.com/teenage-consumer-spending-statistics
2. J. Twenge. *Generation Me: Revised and Updated: Why Today's Young Americans Are More Confident, Assertive, Entitled--and More Miserable Than Ever Before*. Atria Books, 2014.

Chapter 6

1. S.I. Powers, S.T. Hauser, J.M. Schwartz, G.G. Noam, and A.M. Jacobson. "Adolescent Ego Development and Family Interactions: A Structural-Developmental View" in Adolescent Development in the Family: New Directions for Child Development 22. eds. H.D. Grotevant and C.R. Cooper. (San Francisco: Jossey-Bass, 1983).
2. J.E. Marcia, "The Empirical Study of Ego Identity" in Identity and Development: An Interdisciplinary Approach: 67–80, eds. H.A. Bosma, T.L.G. Graafsma, H.D. Grotevant, and D.J. de Levita. (London: Sage, 1984).

Chapter 7

1. David and Linda Bell, "Parental Validation and Support in the Development of Adolescent Daughters" in Adolescent Development in the Family. eds. Harold Grotevant and Catherine Cooper. (San Francisco: Jossey-Bass, 1983).
2. Terri Apter, *Altered Loves: Mothers and Daughters During Adolescence*. (New York: St. Martin's Press, 1990).
3. Daniel Goleman, *Working with Emotional Intelligence*. New York: Bantam. Gottman, John. 1995. *Why Marriages Succeed or Fail and How You Can Make Yours Last*. (New York: Simon & Schuster, 2000).
4. S. Murmen, C. Wright, and G. Kaluzny. "If 'Boys Will Be Boys,' Then Girls Will Be Victims? A Meta-analytic Review of the Research that Relates Masculine Ideology to Sexual Aggression" in Sex Roles: A Journal of Research, 6 (2002): 1–24. D. J. Parrott, A. Zeichner, "Effects of hypermasculinity on physical aggression against women." Psychology of Men & Masculinity, Vol 4(1), Jan [2003]: 70-78.
5. www.investors.com/news/teens-spending-even-more-on-makeup-heres-how-investors-can-benefit
6. J. Snarey, *How Fathers Care for the Next Generation: A Four Decade Study*. Cambridge, Massachusetts: Harvard University Press (1993).

7. J. Pleck, "Paternal Involvement." Pp. 66–107 in The Role of the Father in Child Development. ed. M. Lamb. (New York: Wiley, 1997).

Chapter 8
1. www.pewinternet.org/2015/08/06/teens-technology-and-friendships
2. L.M. Jones, K.J. Mitchell, & D. Finkelhor. (2013). Online harassment in context: Trends from three Youth Internet Safety Surveys (2000, 2005, 2010). Psychology of Violence, 3(1), 53-69.

Chapter 9
1. V. Rideout, U. Foehr, D. Roberts. GENERATION M2: Media in the Lives of 8- to 18-Year-Olds. The Henry J Kaiser Family Foundation, 2010.
2. www.commonsensemedia.org
3. C. Donahue, (Ed.) Family Engagement in the Digital Age: Early Childhood Educators as Media Mentors. Rutledge, 2016.
4. Y.T. Uhls and P.M. Greenfield, (2012). "The Value of Fame: Preadolescent Perceptions of Popular Media and Their Relationship to Future Aspirations," Developmental Psychology, 48(2), 315-326.
5. www.pewinternet.org/2015/04/09/teens-social-media-technology-2015
6. www.pewinternet.org/2015/08/06/teens-technology-and-friendships
7. www.pewinternet.org/2015/08/06/teens-technology-and-friendships
8. Patti M. Valkenburg and Jochen Peter. "Social Consequences of the Internet for Adolescents: A Decade of Research," Current Directions in Psychological Science 18 (1) (2009): 1-5.
9. Jay Giedd. "The Digital Revolution and Adolescent Brain Evolution," Journal of Adolescent Health 51 (2) (2012): 101-105.
10. Twenge, J.M., Joiner, T., Rogers, M., Margin, G.N. "Increases in Depressive Symptoms, Suicide-Related Outcomes, and Suicide Rates Among U.S. Adolescents After 2010 and Links to Increased New Media Screen Time," Clinical Psychological Science, 6 (1) (2018): 3-16.
11. www.puresight.com/Pedophiles/Online-Predators/online-predators-statistics.html
12. Kimberly J. Mitchell and Lisa M. Jones, "Cyberbullying Must Be Studied Within a Broader Peer Victimization Framework," Journal of Adolescent Health 56 (5) (2015): 473-474.
13. Faye Mishna, Alan McLuckie, and Michael Saini, "Real-World Dangers in an Online Reality: A Qualitative Study Examining Online Relationships and Cyber Abuse," Social Work Research 33(2) (2009): 107-118.
14. Kimberly J. Mitchell, Michele L. Ybarra, Lisa M. Jones & Dorothy Espelage, "What Features Make Online Harassment Incidents Upsetting to Youth," Journal of School Violence 3 (2016): 279-301
15. www.apa.org/monitor/2011/06/cheat.aspx. Survey report: http://josephsoninstitute.org/surveys
16. Fred Sandsmark, "Your Cheatin' Heart Doesn't Stand a Chance" in TechWeek, January 2000. www.techweek.com
17. Stephen F. Davis, Patrick F. Drinan, and Tricia Bertram Gallant, T.B., Cheating in School: What We Know and What We Can Do. (Wiley-Blackwell, 2009).
18. E.I. Zurbriggen, Chair, APA Task Force on the Sexualization of Girls, APA Online, press release, February 19, 2007.
19. L. Monique Ward. "Media and Sexualization: State of Empirical Research," The Journal of Sex Research 53 (4-5) (2016): 560-577.
20. Eric W. Owens, Richard J. Behun, Jill C. Manning, Rory C. Reid. "The Impact of Internet Pornography on Adolescents: A Review of the Research," Sexual Addiction & Compulsivity 19 (2012): 99-122.
21. Andrew K. Przybylski and Victoria Nash. "Internet Filtering Technology and Aversive Online Experiences in Adolescents," The Journal of Pediatrics 184 (2017): 215-219.
22. Dahan Boyd, It's Complicated: The Social Lives of Networked Teens. (Yale University Press, 2014).
23. A. Kanner and T. Kasser. eds. Psychology and Consumer Culture: The Struggle for a Good Life in a Materialistic World. American Psychological Association, October 2003.
24. M. Buijzen and P. M. Valkenburg. "The Effects of Television Advertising on Materialism, Parent-Child Conflict, and Unhappiness: A Review of Research" in Applied Developmental Psychology 24 (2003): 437–56.
25. T. Kasser, The High Price of Materialism. (Cambridge: MIT Press, 2002).
26. Jay N. Giedd. "The Digital Revolution and Adolescent Brain Evolution," Journal of Adolescent Health 51 (1) (2013): 101-105.

27. John P. Murray, Barrbara Biggins, Edward Donnerstein, Roy W. Menninger, Michael Rich, and Victor Strasburger. Mayo Clinics Proceedings 86 (8) (2011): 818-820.
28. Isabela Granic, Adam Lobel, Rutger C. M. E. Engels. "The Benefits of Playing Video Games," American Psychologist, 69 (1) (2013): 66-78
29. www.pewinternet.org/2015/08/06/teens-technology-and-friendships
30. S. Lemola, N. Perkinson-Gloor, S. Brand, J.F. Deward-Kaufmann, and A. Grob. "Adolesents' electronic media use at night, sleep disturbance, and depressive symptoms in the Smart Phone age," Journal of Youth and Adolescence, 44 (2) (2015): 405-418.
31. Jerald Block. Editorial: Issues for DSM-V: Internet Addiction. The American Journal of Psychiatry 165(3) (2008): 306-307.
32. A.K. Przybylski and N. Weinstein. "A Large-Scale Test of the Goldilocks Hypothesis," Psychological Science 28 (2) (2017): 204-216.
33. Daniel Goleman, Social Intelligence. (New York: Bantam, 2006).
34. Yalda T. Uhls, Minas Michikyan, Jordan Morris, Debra Garcia, Gary W. Small, Eleni Zgourou, and Patricia M. Greenfield. "Five days at outdoor education camp without screens improves preteen skills with nonverbal emotion cues," Computers in Human Behavior 39 (2014): 387-392.

Chapter 10

1. A. Bartels and S. Zek. "The Neural Basis of Love" in NeuroReport 11, 3 (2000) 829–834.
2. Lisa M. Diamond and David M. Huebner. "Is Good Sex Good for You? Rethinking Sexuality and Health" Social and Personality Psychology Compass 6 (1) (2012): 54-69.
3. G.I. Roisman, W.A. Collins, L. Sroufe, and B. Egeland. "Predictors of Young Adults' Representations of and Behavior in Their Current Romantic Relationships: Prospective Tests of the Prototype Hypothesis" in Attachment and Human Development, 7 (2005); 105–21.
4. www.aap.org/en-us/about-the-aap/aap-press-room/Pages/AAP-Statement-in-Support-of-Transgender-Children-Adolescent-and-Young-Adults.aspx
5. Brian Soller. "Caught in a Bad Romance", Journal of Health and Social Behavior 5 (1) (2014): 56-72.
6. www.cdc.gov/violenceprevention/intimatepartnerviolence/teen_dating_violence.html
7. www.cdc.gov/violenceprevention/intimatepartnerviolence/teen_dating_violence.html
8. www.breakthecycle.org/dating-violence-research/teen-dating-abuse-survey-2006
9. www.breakthecycle.org/dating-violence-research/teen-dating-abuse-survey-2006
10. www.breakthecycle.org/dating-violence-research/teen-dating-abuse-survey-2006
11. Jeff R Temple, Vi D Le, Alexandra Muir, Laurie Goforth, and Amy L. McElhany. "The Need for School-Based Teen Dating Violence Prevention," Journal of Applied Research on Children: Informing Policy for Children at Risk 4 (1), Article 4 (2013). Available at: www.digitalcommonslibrary.tmc.edu/childrenatrisk/vol4/issl/4
12. www.futureswithoutviolence.org/talk-teens-teen-dating-violence

Chapter 11

1. SA Duke, BW Balzer, and KS Steinbeck, "Testosterone and its effects on human male adolescent mood and behavior: a systematic review," Journal of Adolescent Health 55 (3) 2014: 315-322.
2. Jeffrey M. Spielberg, Erika E. Forbes, Cecile D. Ladouceur, Carol M. Worthman, Thomas M. Olino, Neal D. Ryan, Ronald E. Dahl "Pubertal testosterone influences threat-related amygdala–orbitofrontal cortex coupling," Social Cognitive and Affective Neuroscience, 10 (3) (2015): 408–415.
3. Judy Graber. Pubertal timing and the development of psychopathology in adolescence and beyond. Hormones and Behavior 6 (2013): 262–269.
4. Louise Greenspan and Julianna Deardorff. The New Puberty. How to Navigate Early Development in Today's Girls. Rodale Press, 2014.
5. J. Croll, D. Neumark-Sztainer, M. Story, and M. Ireland. "Prevalence and Risk and Protective Factors Related to Disordered Eating Behaviors Among Adolescents: Relationship to Gender and Ethnicity," Journal of Adolescent Health, 31 (2002): 166–75.
6. Jasmin Langdon-Daly & Lucy Serpell. "Protective factors against disordered eating in family systems; a systematic review of research," Journal of Eating Disorders 5 (12) (2017): 1-15
7. R.W. Blum, "Mothers' Influence on Teen Sex: Connections that Promote Postponing Sexual Intercourse," Center for Adolescent Health and Development. (University of Minnesota, 2002).
8. J. Santelli and M. Ott. "Abstinence-only Education Policies and Programs: A Position Paper for the Society of Adolescent Medicine," Journal of Adolescent Health: 38 (2006): 83–7.

9. Trenholm C, et al., Impacts of Four Title V, Section 510 Abstinence Education Programs Final Report. Princeton, NJ: Mathematic Policy Research; submitted to U.S. Dept. Health & Human Services, Assistant Secretary for Planning and Evaluation, 2007.

10. JC Abma and GM Martinez. "Sexual Activity and Contraceptive Use Among Teenagers in The United States, 2011-2015. National Health Statistics Reports, No. 104, June 22, 2017.

11. Kathryn Kost and Stanley Henshaw. "U.S. Teenage Pregnancies, Births and Abortions, 2010: National and State Trends by Age, Race and Ethnicity," Guttmacher Institute (2014): 1-29

Chapter 12

1. David R. Topor, Susan P. Keane, and Terri L. Shelton, "Parent involvement and student academic performance: A multiple mediational analysis," Journal of Prevention and Intervention in the Community, 38 (3) (2010): 183-97.

2. C. Spera, "A Review of the Relationship Among Parenting Practices, Parenting Styles, and Adolescent School Achievement." Educational Psychology Review, 17 (2) (2005): 125-146.

3. S. Luthar and B. Becker. "Privileged But Pressured? A Study of Affluent Youth" in Child Development, 73 (5) (2002): 1593-610.

4. Carol Dweck, *Mindset: The New Psychology of Success.* (New York: Random House, 2006).

5. C. Blair. "'Treating a Toxin to Learning," Scientific American Mind, Sept/Oct 2012.

6. Jeylan T. Mortimer. "The Benefits and Risks of Adolescent Employment," Prevention Research 17 (2) (2010): 8-ll.

7. Astin, A. What Matters in College: Four Critical Years Revisited. (San Francisco: Jossey-Bass, 1991).

8. J.A. Durlak, R.P. Weissberg, A.B. Dymnicki, R.D. Taylor, K.B. Schellinger. "The impact of enhancing students' social and emotional learning: a meta-analysis of school-based universal interventions, Child Development 82 (1) 2011: 405-32.

9. Laura Kastner and Jennifer Wyatt. *The Launching Years.* (New York: Three Rivers Press, 2002).

Chapter 13

1. Statistics on teen substance use come from the Youth Risk Behavior Surveillance System (YRBSS): www.cdc.gov/healthyyouth/data/yrbs/index.htm?s_cid=hy-homepage

2. Michelle L. Macy, Patrick M. Carter, C. Raymond Bingham, Rebecca M. Cunningham, Gary L. Freed. "Potential Distractions and Unsafe Driving Behaviors Among Drivers of 1- to 12-Year-Old Children." Academic Pediatrics, 2014; 14 (3): 279-286.

3. www.drugabuse.gov/news-events/news-releases/2016/12/teen-substance-use-shows-promising-decline

4. L. Steinberg, "Risk-taking in Adolescence: New Perspectives from Brain and Behavioral Science" in Current Directions in Psychological Science, 16 (2007): 55–9.

5. Deborah Gorman-Smith, "Urban Neighborhoods, Families, and Juvenile Delinquency" in The Prevention Researcher, 15 (1) (2008): 17–20.

Chapter 14

1. Felitti, V.J. et al. "Relationship of Childhood Abuse and Household Dysfunction to Many of the Leading Causes of Death in Adults: The Adverse Childhood Experiences (ACE) Study." American Journal of Preventive Medicine 14, (4) (1998): 245–58.

2. Duncan, L., J.D. Coatsworth, and M. Greenberg. "A Model of Mindful Parenting: Implications for Parent-child Relationships and Prevention Research." Clinical Child and Family Psychology Review 12, (3) (2009): 255–70.

Resources

Parenting Basics

Kastner, L. and J. Wyatt. *The Seven-Year Stretch: How Families Work Together to Grow Through Adolescence.* New York: Houghton-Mifflin, 1997.

Kastner, L. and Russell, K. (Contributor). *Wise Minded Parenting: 7 Essentials for Raising Successful Tweens + Teens,* ParentMap, 2013.

Lythcott-Haims, Julie. *How to Raise an Adult: Break Free of the Overparenting Trap and Prepare Your Kid for Success,* Henry Holt & Co, 2015.

Mogel, Wendy. *The Blessing of a Skinned Knee: Using Jewish Teachings to Raise Self-Reliant Children,* Scribner, 2008.

Siegel, Daniel and Mary Hartzell. *Parenting from the Inside Out: How a Deeper Self-Understanding Can Help You Raise Children Who Thrive,* Tarcher/Penguin, 2004.

The Brain and Emotion

Siegel, Daniel J. and Bryson, Tina P. *The Yes Brain: How to Cultivate Courage, Curiosity, and Resilience in Your Child,* Bantam, 2018.

Siegel, Daniel J., *Brainstorm: The Power and Purpose of the Teenage Brain,* TarcherPerigee, 2014.

Harvey, Pat and Rathbone, B.H *Parenting a Teen Who Has Intense Emotions: DBT Skills to Help Your Teen Navigate Emotional and Behavioral Challenges,* New Harbinger Publ, 2015.

McGonigal, Kelly. *The Willpower Instinct: How Self-Control Works, Why it Matters, and What You Can Do to Get More of It.* Gildan Media, 2012.

Gender Issues: Girls

Damour, Lisa. *Untangled: Guiding Teenage Girls Through the Seven Transitions into Adulthood,* Ballantine Books, 2016.

Catherine Steiner-Adair and Lisa Sjostrom. *Full of Ourselves: A Wellness Program to Advance Girl Power, Health, and Leadership.* Teachers College Press, 2005.

Gender Issues: Boys

Thompson, Michael. *It's a Boy! Your Son's Development from Birth to Age 18,* Random House, 2008.

Pollock, William. *Real Boys: Rescuing Our Sons from the Myths of Boyhood.* Owl Books, 1999.

Dating and Sexuality

Geltman, Joani. *A Survival Guide to Parenting Teens: Talking to Your Kids About Sexting, Drinking, Drugs, and Other Things That Freak You Out,* AMACOM, 2014.

Huegel, Kelly. *GLBTQ: The Survival Guide for Gay, Lesbian, Bisexual, Transgender, and Questioning Teens,* Free Spirit Publishing, 2011.

Lang, Amy. *Dating Smarts – What Every Teen Needs to Date, Relate or Wait*, Birds + Bees + Kids, LLC, 2014.

Langford, Jo. *Spare Me "The Talk"!: A Guy's Guide to Sex, Relationships and Growing Up*, ParentMap, 2015.

Langford, Jo. *Spare Me "The Talk"!: A Girl's Guide to Sex, Relationships, and Growing Up*, ParentMap, 2016.

Social Development

Borba, M. *Unselfie: Why Empathetic Kids Succeed in Our All-About-Me World*, Touchstone, 2017.

Greene, R. W. *Raising Human Beings: Creating a Collaborative Partnership With Your Child*, Scribner, 2017.

Media and Technology Issues

boyd, danah. *It's Complicated: The Social Lives of Networked Teens*, Yale University Press, 2014.

Gold, J. and Burch, T. *Screen-Smart Parenting: How to Find Balance and Benefit in Your Child's Use of Social Media, Apps, and Digital Devices*, Guilford, 2014.

Steiner-Adair, C. *The Big Disconnect: Protecting Childhood and Family Relationships in the Digital Age*. Harper Collins, 2013.

Turkle, S. *Alone Together: Why We Expect More from Technology and Less from Each Other*, Basic Books, 2012.

Uhls, Y. *Media Moms & Digital Dads: A Fact-Not-Fear Approach to Parenting in the Digital Age*, Taylor & Francis, 2015.

Stress Reduction

Bradley, M. *Crazy-Stressed: Saving Today's Overwhelmed Teens With Love, Laughter, and the Science of Resilience*, AMACOM, 2017.

Saltzman, A. *A Still Quiet Place for Teens: A Mindfulness Workbook to Ease Stress and Difficult Emotions*, Instant Help, 2016.

Seligman, Martin. *Flourish: A Visionary New Understanding of Happiness and Well-Being*, Atria Books, 2012.

Vo, Dzung X. *The Mindful Teen: Powerful Skills to Help You Handle Stress One Moment at a Time*, Instant Help, 2015.

Williams, Mark and Penman, Danny. *Mindfulness: An Eight-Week Plan for Finding Peace in a Frantic World*, Rodale Books, 2012

Index

About ParentMap

ParentMap is a media company that inspires, supports, and connects a growing community of wise-minded parents by publishing intelligent, trusted and thought-leading content to equip them for their essential role as their child's first and most important teacher. ParentMap's unique social-venture business model drives its vision and day-to-day operations, ensuring that publication readers and website visitors are given the most current information related to early learning, fun adventures, child health and development, and parenting. In all of its work and through all of its resources and publishing channels, ParentMap is dedicated to providing outstanding editorial content, advocating for children and families, and contributing to community.

Visit us at *parentmap.com*.

Other ParentMap titles:

Spare Me 'The Talk'!: A Guy's Guide to Sex, Relationships, and Growing Up
By Jo Langford, M.A.

Spare Me 'The Talk'!: A Girl's Guide to Sex, Relationships, and Growing Up
By Jo Langford, M.A.

Wise-Minded Parenting: 7 Essentials for Raising Successful Tweens + Teens
By Laura S. Kastner, Ph.D. with Kristen A. Russell

Getting to Calm, The Early Years: Cool-Headed Strategies for Raising Happy, Caring, and Independent Three- to Seven-Year-Olds
By Laura S. Kastner, Ph.D.

Beyond Smart: Boosting Your Child's Social, Emotional and Academic Potential By Linda Morgan

Northwest Kid Trips By Lora Shinn

ParentMap books are available at special discounts when purchased in bulk for premiums and sales promotions, as well as for fundraisers or educational use. Contact *books@parentmap.com* for more information.

About the Authors

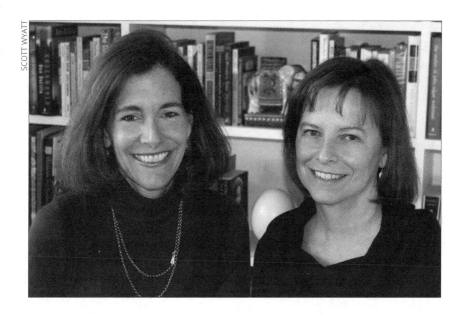

Laura S. Kastner, Ph.D., is a clinical professor of psychiatry and behavioral sciences at the University of Washington who lectures widely on adolescence and family behavior. She is a psychologist and mother of two. **Jennifer Wyatt, Ph.D.,** contributes to parenting publications and has taught at the college and high school levels. She is a writer, mother of four, and grandparent of three. They are the authors of *The Launching Years: Strategies for Parenting from Senior Year to College Life* and *The Seven-Year Stretch: How Families Work Together to Grow Through Adolescence.* Additionally, Dr. Kastner has authored *Wise-Minded Parenting: 7 Essentials for Raising Successful Tweens & Teens* (Kristen Russell, contributor) and *Getting to Calm, The Early Years: Cool-Headed Strategies for Raising Happy, Caring and Independent 3- to 7-Year-Olds.*